Atrial Fibrillation

My Heart, The Doctors
and me

AN INVESTIGATIVE REPORT BY AN INQUISITIVE PATIENT

OTHER WORKS BY THE AUTHOR

THE RIGHT APPROACH
***
MOVE IN & MOVE UP
***
THE BIG BUCK AND THE NEW BUSINESS
BREED
***
PEOPLE AND PROFITS
***
PROS AND CONS OF
MANAGEMENT CONSULTANTS
***
ON THE JOB
A NATIONALLY SYNDICATED
BUSINESS COLUMN

Atrial Fibrillation

My Heart, The Doctors and me

AN INVESTIGATIVE REPORT BY AN INQUISITIVE PATIENT

by

E. A. Butler

Edited and Introduced
by
John F. Mullane, M.D., Ph.D., J.D.

King of Hearts Publishing Company, Inc.
458 Edith Avenue
Salt Lake City, Utah 84111

Copyright © 2000 by E. A. Butler

King of Hearts Publishing Company, Inc.
458 Edith Avenue, Salt Lake City, Utah 84111
e-mail: pbjet@aol.com
Telephone: 801-484-1183

E. A. Butler: e-mail adb2530@ix.netcom.com
Telephone: 518-793-4375; Fax: 518-793-3300

ISBN 0-9675203-0-4
LIBRARY OF CONGRESS CATALOG CARD NUMBER:99-91049

Printed in the United States of America
0987654321

My gratitude goes to my wife, Ann, without whose help, understanding, and punctuation this work could not have been accomplished and, needless to say, to the many doctors, health writers, research scientists, and patients with atrial fibrillation/flutter for making this work possible.

CONTENTS

FOREWORD

Diligent research for this book has proven that millions of people with atrial fibrillation (700 thousand newly diagnosed cases each year) are frantically searching for any encouraging information about this elusive and not so well understood arrhythmia of the heart. As one of those, I've attempted to educate myself on how I can live a more productive life without its psychological or physical burdens.

I've come to believe that many doctors are overwhelmed with constant and conflicting information and questionable sales approaches from some pharmaceutical companies.

The patient often assumes doctors are able to absorb this confusing information, separate it in a highly structured form, and apply what's right without further question.

Today's patients are exposed to differing opinions, media medical hype, and heavily advertised miracle treatments.

FOREWORD

I've evaluated volumes of material and selected those I think are the most helpful and informative.

This book deals with me as a patient, what I have experienced and learned and how I ultimately cut down my fibrillations from as many as three a week to just two a year, thereby dramatically lessening my chances of crippling strokes.

A glossary of medical terms, a list of web pages, and a bibliography that includes newspapers, books and medical periodicals, are included in the back of the book.

This book is not intended to replace professional medical advice. Only a doctor can diagnose and treat medical problems.

My thanks to Dr. John Mullane for his repeated readings and checking for mistakes in the use of medical references.

E.A.B.

INTRODUCTION

About a year ago, my friend, E. A. Butler, came to me with several questions about the technical use of words and phrases in a book he was working on about atrial fibrillation.

We discussed his questions in great detail and later I found his approach to the subject fascinating, particularly because at the time I was unaware of any published book from a patient's viewpoint.

I can understand the perplexities of the millions of people who suffer this malady. It's one of the more exasperating and elusive problems in the cardiovascular world.

I suggested I might help him best by reviewing and editing all the medical terminologies used in the book, yet not interfering with his perspective of cardiovascular disease.

If anyone could write a book about this subject, I knew he could. His professional research skills were developed while writing a syndicated business column for the Chicago Tribune-New York Daily News.

He concentrated on dissecting American industry. This experience helped him evaluate and tie together the healthcare industry's approach to atrial fibrillation and how it's handled.

I like his present work because it is in the same concise vein as were his other books and columns.

His extensive exposure to the drug industry in his role as a management and executive search consultant served me well.

As I built American Home Product's pharmaceutical research facility in Princeton, NJ, he personally recruited the Vice President of Research and all research department directors. He also assisted me in evaluating the managerial skills of several research and development department heads, including Vice Presidents of Clinical Research and Medical Marketing.

During business meetings and many rounds of golf, I've observed his insatiable desire for knowledge and his mastery at analyzing people. We often discussed the drugs I was developing such as Inderal®, Coumadin®, Cozaar® Cardiolite®, Premarin® and Lodine®, many of which are mentioned in this book.

He's interviewed many of America's academic leaders in cardiovascular medicine in the course of this work for me and other clients. These prior contacts facilitated his acquisition of knowledge from America's premier heart specialists. His description of personal experiences highlights the uncertainty that exists when the science of a disease is still evolving and ideal therapies are not yet available.

As he describes the nuisance of his arrhythmia attacks, the reader not only learns about many of the medical approaches to this condition, but also experiences his confusion, frustration, and reactions to information provided by physicians and fellow disease sufferers.

E. A. Butler has provided personal interpretations and criticisms of the medical therapeutics for this potentially serious disorder that should prove to be useful for readers interested in disorders of the heart.

John F. Mullane, M.D., Ph.D., J.D.

Atrial Fibrillation

My Heart, The Doctors
and me

AN INVESTIGATIVE REPORT BY AN INQUISITIVE PATIENT

I

A BIG SURPRISE

This August day was one of those near perfect days in the foothills of the beautiful Adirondacks.

Inside the impressive brick building the cardiologist's office was bustling with activities. I was there for my annual physical. This visit was part of a regular routine I'd practiced for more than thirty-five years. Fortunately for me, with only a few minor exceptions (an occasional "skipped" heart beat from too much coffee), the examinations had always come out great.

Most often, I left the doctor's office with the feeling that all was right with the world and hopefully I could look forward to another healthy year. I could think of no reason why the upcoming examination would not be the same.

I was now enjoying, as the cliché goes, the Golden Years, and this morning's visit was at a time when every healthy day meant more than usual to me.

As I sat quietly in the outer office I reflected on the growing of my children. I recalled I'd not been able to spend the time with them as I now wish I had.

During that period, my absence seemed perfectly justifiable. The company I had founded four decades earlier was engaged in corporate consulting. This occupation required traveling about seventy-five percent of the time.

It was worse for me because some years before, in 1973, I'd moved my family from the tumultuous turmoil of New York City to a small and peaceful upstate town. I wanted them to benefit from the freedom of movement I'd enjoyed when I was a boy in a similar town in North Carolina. At that time in the Big Apple, children couldn't walk or ride their bikes to school or go unescorted to the homes of friends. It was no longer safe.

Because of the demands of my business, and the termination of Mohawk Airline flights to upstate New York, this move required me to remain in the city during the week and for the most part be home only on weekends. Now, though my children were married and living out west, my semi-retirement would enable my wife and me to visit their homes more frequently and hopefully I could get to know them better. I wanted in a big way to make up for the time I was absent when they were young and growing into adolescence.

Quite suddenly my daydreaming was interrupted

when a young nurse, frocked in a white coat, opened a door leading to the inner sanctum and called my first name as though she were addressing a child in the first grade. I obediently followed her into one of several small rooms that lined the narrow hall. There I was weighed and then told to remove my clothing to the waist. When she left the room I found a magazine I could peruse till the cardiologist entered. After appropriate greetings, he routinely performed a blood pressure test and informed me the results were much the same as last year. The reading was 140/90. That, he said, was borderline hypertension, though not unreasonably high for my age.

This information was welcomed. After all, I was 68 and knew that one must expect the body to change somewhat with age. The doctor continued checking my heart and lungs with his stethoscope. After several probes he reported it all sounded normal. My pulse was 75, and my lungs were clear. After all this, my usual office apprehension had gradually subsided.

Twenty minutes later he left the room. His young assistant appeared again and beckoned me to follow her into the "monster room", technically known as the stress test room. In there was an uncomplicated looking exercise machine with a large readout screen attached at eye level and a treadmill for one to walk on at varying degrees of incline. When the contraption was occupied and running, it enabled the technician to chart what was going on inside the user's heart. This machine was no stranger to me. I had had the test many times before as part of the annual examination.

As I lay on the table the nurse began lubricating the spots where disks with wires to the tester would be placed. This helped them make better contact with the body. I guessed there were at least ten attached to me, including the ones just above the ankles.

With the wires hanging from my body I carefully stepped on the treadmill and the young nurse started the machine. It all began so very innocently.

Without belaboring the point, she now watched both me and the screen as I slowly began the ten minute trek.

At least two minutes passed before she asked how I felt. When I responded, "Fine," she sped the thing up while increasing the incline. This routine went on for several more minutes till the wall clock said I'd been walking this stationary hike for about nine minutes. Suddenly she abruptly stared at me and appeared startled. She inquired if I was all right. I told her I was and aside from becoming slightly tired all else was the same as in previous tests. Moments later she again looked up at me then hustled out of the room.

It was less than thirty seconds before she was back with the doctor. Without looking in my direction they both stared at the still active display. Seconds later, the doctor asked, "You okay?" Again I told them I felt nothing different. I was indeed beginning to wonder what the flurry of this unusual activity was all about. He then asked if I could keep it up for another minute. "No problem," I bragged smartly. When the minute passed the doctor slowed the treadmill till it stopped and held my arm as I got off. "Do you feel dizzy?" he asked. Once again I assured him nothing had changed. He directed me to lie on the table while he monitored the screen. The receptors were still attached to me.

Several minutes passed before he began massaging my neck just below the angle of my jaw. I later learned he was stimulating a sensitive nerve near the carotid artery on the right side of my neck to return my heart beat to normal. It was something I'd not experienced before.

Obviously today things were rotten in Denmark, or more precisely, in my heart. A few more minutes passed before he told me I could sit up while the technician removed the disks. As I did, I hastily inquired, "What the devil was that all about?"

"You've experienced an *atrial flutter,*" he answered quietly. "It's stopped now and your heart is back in sinus rhythm."

"Back in what?" I asked rather excitedly.

"You had an *arrhythmia,*" he said dryly. These two medical terms were new to me. Like most Americans I was quite familiar with cholesterol, high blood pressure, stroke, bypass and transplant surgery.

Today, one must be deaf, dumb, blind or living in a hole not to know about them, but not these new words, *"atrial"* or *"arrhythmia."*

My mind was racing hard to comprehend just what he was saying to me. I could barely hear him. "It's not life threatening," he said quietly. I tried hard to control my outward composure.

In this brief state of confusion, I anxiously asked "Who gets this thing? How can something be wrong with my heart and not be life threatening?"

"It most often comes along with age," he answered. "As far as I can tell you haven't any underlying heart disease." He suggested I get dressed and come to his office so he could tell me more.

He left the room to return to the patient he'd abruptly left when the technician sought him out.

In no time at all I was waiting in his office at the end of the corridor and trying hard to be patient....Boy, was this beautiful August day ruined, I thought.

Finally the good doctor entered his office and casually sat down on the edge of his desk. In his left hand he had a plastic replica of a human heart. The heart was sectioned to come apart. I listened attentively as he pointed out the various chambers. He explained the function of the right and left atria (upper heart chambers), and the right and left ventricles (lower heart chambers). He then illustrated how the blood returns to the heart from the body through the vena cava (final large vein collecting my blood). It then enters the right atrium and is pumped through the tricuspid valve (a channel to prevent regurgitation of blood) into the right ventricle and from there through the pulmonic valve into the pulmonary artery to the lungs where it receives oxygen. The oxygenated blood then returns from the lungs through the pulmonary veins and on to the left atrium and ventricle. The mitral valve (like a partition) separates the left atrium and ventricle. When the left atrium is full the blood is pumped through the mitral valve into the left ventricle. It then exits the left ventricle and flows through the aortic valve and then through the aorta to the various organs in the body. He had tried very hard with his chart and plastic heart to explain what makes my heart function properly.

"Your problem," he said "is in the *sinus node*. That's where the electrical impulse begins to make the heart function. It's located at the top of the right atrium. It initiates an *electrical impulse* that flows over the right and left atria making them contract. When the charge reaches the atrioventricular node (he pointed this node out on the model), it's delayed slightly. It then continues down other routes to the right and left ventricles. There, it spreads over the ventricles till they contract, resulting in a pumping action that sends oxygenated blood through the aorta and out through the body."

Whew, I thought, what a mouthful. It was indeed all Greek to me.

As I tried to put together what he was saying, I envisioned the sinus node like a spark plug in my car. When an auto's spark ignites the gas, it explodes and drives the piston that turns the wheels that make the car move. I decided the body functions were somewhat like a car. I was well aware how important a car's spark plugs are. I knew that when a plug shorts to the engine block, instead of the spark following its normal path the motor will run, but it will run rough. As the saying goes, "It ain't hitting on all cylinders."

Under my stressed circumstances I was glad to have grasped as much of his explanation as I did. I then implored him to explain *atrial flutter*. I recalled his words were like a lighting strike to my brain when I first got off the treadmill.

"With atrial flutter," he continued "the atrium contracts quite rapidly and usually at a different speed than the ventricles. Typically, the ventricular rate is half the atrial rate." To me, this all sounded more serious than he was making it out to be.

The cardiologist's accelerated lesson on my heart was fast coming to an end. He began to move from his desk to the door and as he walked he told me he wanted me to wear a Holter Monitor for twenty-four hours. I followed him back to the stress test room and the same assistant hooked me up to a portable contraption.

For twenty-four hours this gadget would constantly record the activities of my heart on a cassette tape. When analyzed, it would tell the doctor just how well my heart was performing under all conditions. Also, the technician said, with this procedure in the next twenty-four hours, they could tell how many, if any, of these strange new *episodes* I'd had.

When I arrived home, I completely unburdened myself to my wife with all the details of my visit with the doctor. With her typically calm encouragement I tried to accept all that the doctor had told me with a positive outlook.

As I thought over the new monitoring procedure I hoped above all I could follow the nurse's instruction on how to successfully use the recorder. I so wanted the results to be accurate. Also, I was determined to continue doing all the work I'd normally do around the house, though when I was leaving the office, I asked the doctor what limits of physical exertion I'd best observe, and how else I could help myself. He answered quite casually, "Don't chase any bears!" I hastily concluded it didn't take a genius to figure that remark out. Apparently it was my exertion on the treadmill that had precipitated the *flutter* and excessive exercise could produce another *episode*.

I was sure the tone of his voice was deliberate. He wanted to reassure me he didn't believe my new malady was as bad as I pessimistically perceived it to be. After all, I assured myself, I'd been informed over the years by both my old New York City physician, and this doctor, that my heart was comparable to a healthy bull's. Now this *flutter* business had appeared and jarred me off my pins.

Nevertheless, I concluded it would be foolish to stack the fireplace wood under the shed during this hot August day.

For the remainder of the afternoon my mind was preoccupied as I labored much harder than usual. I fiddled around in my wife's rose garden, then quickly swept our long black driveway. As a rule I left the grass cutting for our yard man, though today when I completed my other chores, I mowed the lawn. I'd been deliberately looking for physical challenges to prove to myself there was nothing really wrong with my body. As I moved around the yard I kept fantasizing how, come tomorrow, when the results of the portable gadget were read, the doctor would tell me that I was okay and that his office machine was out of order. I had heard this does occasionally happen.

Time passed at a snail's pace.

The following day about two pm I anxiously showed up at his office and, again, waited for someone to unhook me from the damn contraption. It had been quite cumbersome to wear, and worse, it was always in the way. During the night it woke me each time I turned over to find a more comfortable sleeping position.

Eventually, another assistant rescued me from the crowded waiting room. Again she called my name loud enough to be heard in the street. For reasons I was not quite sure of, I wasn't anxious to let the world know why I was there, and why I was wearing this strange looking Walkman. It may have had something to do with male ego. Fortunately, the only patient I knew in the waiting room was not a close friend.

Again, I followed the nurse. She unhooked me and hurriedly left the room. I presumed she was rushing the recording to the doctor. In twenty minutes or so he arrived and casually informed me I'd experienced another two episodes over the previous twenty-four hours. That really shook me. I'd had no symptoms and was totally unaware that anything unusual was going on inside my heart. I couldn't help but wonder if these things had been happening in the past without any awareness to me, and if so, what caused them. The thought of silent episodes made me feel quite helpless and threatened since my heart at any time might suddenly misfire and I wouldn't know how to deal with it. At the moment I wanted to shout to the doctor, "WHAT THE HELL CONSTITUTES AN EMERGENCY WITH THIS THING."

When my cardiologist's conference began, he said he wanted me to start taking 180 mg of Isoptin® (verapamil hydrochloride.) When I asked what it was, he said it was a calcium-channel blocker. That meant absolutely nothing to me so I asked him to explain. "This drug should, by all accounts, lower your blood pressure." It was then I first realized there might be a relationship between high blood pressure and the electrical abnormality in my heart.

"Hopefully," he added, "lowering your pressure might stop you from having further episodes." I became more encouraged with this news though I worried a bit about his use of, "it should" and "hopefully." Regardless, I thought, maybe our much maligned pharmaceutical industry had a miracle drug that would make my heart function properly.

II

DRUGS AND MORE DRUGS

I took my prescribed pill faithfully each day from August to January. During this period I was without further episodes. I was just beginning to think I was home free when it happened again.

Early one very cold January morning, while walking my dog in the park next to my home, I must have been exerting myself more than I realized. The temperature was 30 below zero. In the foothills of the Adirondacks this temperature is not terribly unusual at this time of year.

Twenty minutes or so after returning home, I had what I thought was a mild bout of indigestion. For whatever reason, I unconsciously felt my pulse and detected a very erratic beat. As the arrhythmia continued my mind was also vibrating as though an explosion had just happened in my ear. It was Sunday and I was in a quandary about calling my doctor at his residence.

During the past four months I'd done some research on *atrial flutter* and had learned that out of four million souls with ventricular or atrial arrhythmia, my malady was generally classified as "paroxysmal" or *"lone" atrial flutter.* A publication put out by the American Heart Association confirmed that some 302,000 souls in 1995 were admitted to hospitals with *arrhythmias.* As near as I could tell, of that number, there were 46,000 deaths. It appeared most of these deaths resulted from ventricular fibrillation which obviously was much more life threatening.

I also obtained another interesting opinion from one of my close friends, Dr. John Mullane, who had been Executive Vice President for Research & Development, including Medical Affairs, for the Ayerst Division of American Home Products. He is a leading, twenty-five year research and development pharmaceutical executive who has been with two international drug developers (Ayerst and DuPont-Merck). Dr. Mullane was associated with the development and growth of three major cardiovascular drugs: Inderal®, the first beta-blocker; Coumadin®, a leading blood thinning drug; and Cozaar®, the first angiotensin II blocking drug for hypertension.

He firmly believes, at any given time, there are some 15,000,000 people walking around with undiagnosed cases of arrhythmias. "These people either don't know they have the problem, do not recognize the symptoms to be serious, or have an unfortunate case of denial. Often the diagnosis is made and therapy is considered when the condition grows unbearable or when the arrhythmia is detected during a routine check-up, such as occurred with you. Sadly, in some cases the arrhythmia is fatal," he grimly added.

I was quite happy to have it confirmed that in the absence of any underlying heart disease, atrial flutter, usually in itself, isn't likely to do me in.

Paroxysmal sounded horrible enough on its own. To me, it conjured up the same fear as the word cancer, though literally, it simply means spasm or "intermittent," but to my dismay I also learned there was an increased, though very minor, possibility of a stroke during an episode.

A lot of my concerns stemmed from my family history. My brother had suffered a severe stroke at 74 and my sister began having TIAs (mini strokes or transient ischemic attacks affecting the brain) at about 65.

On further research I discovered the risk of stroke is less with flutter than with fibrillation since the atria contract more vigorously with flutter. This was enough to continue focusing my serious attention toward more detailed research.

Finally, I mustered my courage to disturb my doctor during his much deserved day of rest. Unfortunately his answering service said he was out of town. They referred me to another associate who was covering his patients during his absence. When my call was returned, the covering doctor seemed quite casual and suggested that if the episode lasted more than twenty-four hours I should go to the emergency room and arrange for "*cardioversion.*" Of course, I jested to myself, he meant, if I hadn't had a stroke in the meantime.

He also suggested I not stress my heart by walking again in this sub-zero weather. I mused at his cautious, but unnecessary warning.

Cardioversion, to me, was another unfamiliar medical word that was now in play. When I inquired what this was all about, he explained that they used a machine that produced a mild electrical shock to the heart, similar to the machine used by rescue squads and firemen to restart the heart of heart attack victims, but with a lower dose of electricity for the atrial flutter/fibrillation patients.

Two disks are used, one placed on the left side of your chest and the other on the right. An electrical charge is arced across the chest. This charge usually returns the heart to its normal beat (*sinus rhythm*). It sounded to me like a very complicated and unpleasant procedure. The casualness of his conversation disturbed me enough that I decided to seek a second opinion from a cardiologist whom I knew who was affiliated with a major teaching hospital in Utah.

It was there that I learned that cardioversion works sometime and at others it doesn't. I concluded its really no better than drugs for atrial fibrillation.

III

OTHER
EXPERTS

A few days later I phoned Doctor Jeffrey A. Anderson, who was then Professor of Medicine and Chief of Cardiology at LDS Hospital in Salt Lake City, to make an appointment. Several years before, I'd gotten to know him through my pharmaceutical management consulting activities and knew he was recognized as an excellent cardiologist. He had given me a book he'd edited titled, *"Modern Management of Acute Myocardial Infarction In the Community Hospital."* It was still among my books, though I'd never read it. At that time I had been in excellent health with a normal heart and therefore, like most people without problems, had little or no interest in the details of the subject. I remembered he had said it was sold mostly to cardiologists and hospitals for $95.00 a copy. Now, like most people with their own maladies, I'd developed a much keener interest. As I skimmed through the chapter dealing with *arrhythmia*, I concluded the author of this section seemed to believe that *lone atrial flutter* was something of a medical nuisance. This revelation left me somewhat confused.

To me it was more than just a nuisance. From what research I had done to date, it appeared that other experts felt it was indeed more than just a nuisance. I had learned from my cursory examination of multiple documents from various medical publications dealing with the heart that atrial flutter could convert to atrial fibrillation. I didn't know if this had happened with me but it was a reason for concern.

Atrial fibrillation was responsible for approximately 34% of serious hospital visits for arrhythmia and it was to a high degree significantly associated with morbidity and death. Stroke was one of its leading complications.

Many of the published papers from these creditable sources seemed to have upgraded this problem from a mere nuisance that required mundane attention to one that required a more serious approach.

Jeff's busy schedule prevented me from seeing him until January. When I did see him, he reviewed the electrocardiogram from my primary doctor, then directed one of his assistants to give me a routine examination. When it was over, he spent a bit of time reinforcing what I had learned from him in the earlier phone conversation.

However, he suggested, that to help my peace of mind I see a specialist in the atrial flutter/fibrillation field. This was the first time I had heard there was such a speciality. Had I known, I would have gone directly to one. It was exactly what I originally wanted to do.

He gave me the names of two cardiologists whose reputations, he said, were among the best. One was in Cleveland, Ohio and the other in Northern California.

Because of his proximity, I chose the Cleveland specialist. Unfortunately the earliest appointment I could arrange was the 12th of June, for me a long time away. In the meantime I verified my new specialist's credentials in several reference books and his excellent background made me feel better despite the delay.

Shortly after arriving at his office in June, I gave a copy of the original EKG's I'd brought from my doctor's office to his nurse/assistant. She introduced me to the electrophysiologist who prepared me for an echocardiographic exam. She explained that it enabled them to actually see the heart and how its various chambers functioned. It took about an hour. When I returned to the doctor's office, I broke out the list of questions I'd previously prepared and began interrogating him. Thankfully, he was most patient. He had, as the saying goes, "a real bedside manner." He slowly and carefully answered all my questions from the list I had prepared ahead of time. He drew pictures of just what he envisioned my heart was up to, then explained all the current alternatives.

One of them was a relatively new procedure called "*Cardiac Radiofrequency Ablation.*" When he described it, it made cardioversion sound tame. He explained that under optimum operating room conditions a very thin flexible wire is placed in a vein of an arm or leg and advanced to the right *atrium* of the heart. The electrical conducting system is interrupted or blocked by a small burn made by the wire at a spot in the heart the electrophysiologist has previously identified. This procedure most often stops the chaotic electrical impulses in the atria from reaching the ventricles and effectively slows the heart back to its normal rhythm.

Shortly after recuperation, medications can usually be stopped, except for blood thinners that still could be necessary. He added that the procedure involves a twenty-four to forty-eight hour stay in the hospital with a quick return to full activity (about two weeks). For the most part the *ablation* is regarded as experimental though he said that one day it might provide a cure for atrial flutter.

In spite of its current experimental status, I decided then and there I'd look into this further. If I found it would, indeed, get rid of the condition once and for all, I'd go for it.

Ironically, soon after I returned home, while visiting a new neighbor, I quite accidentally learned his wife had had a successful ablation a couple of years earlier. When I discussed this with her she explained she had experienced arrhythmias since early childhood. I was glad to know someone could have them for that long and not have a disabling stroke or die, though she did explain that her quality of life had been diminished, if only psychologically.

Very shortly after learning of the new ablation technique, she had begun a thorough investigation. Fortunately for me she still had in her possession a number of articles she'd obtained from various sources. I read them diligently. They were useful in helping me to decide that I wanted to explore this relatively new technique further.

One of the articles was from the September 1994 *Reader's Digest* titled, *WHEN THE HEART MISFIRES.* However, it only covered *ventricular* fibrillation, and was my first of many clues that atrial flutter and ventricular fibrillation were two entirely different maladies, even though the two heart chambers depend on the same electrical impulse from the *sinus node.* It sounded to me as if the latter was more serious because of underlying heart disease.

In what seemed like an eternity, but was only a

week, I received a letter from Cleveland enclosing a copy of the echocardiographic report to my doctor. I decided it was more official than his consoling words when I had visited his Cleveland office. The word "normal" ran throughout the pages next to all the criteria discussing the condition of my heart. Reading them made me feel good. However, his letter reminded me he'd inquired several times if I had ever been on a beta-blocker. It was now clear to me why the questions.

In his letter to my doctor he suggested, "A beta-blocker might provide additional benefit by decreasing *adrenergic* tone which could aggravate the *arrhythmia.*" His words struck me as though they were straight from God. After all he was the specialist in this field. While I really didn't know just what *"adrenergic"* meant, I decided that if a beta-blocker would stop it from aggravating my heart, I was all for it.

Quite by coincidence I was familiar with this beta-blocker. One of my old consulting clients, American Home Products, was, for many years, its sole licensed producer for the United States. The drug, Propranolol (the generic name for beta-blockers), had been discovered in England by ICI Chemicals. It is one of the world's largest selling medications. In the mid'80s American Home Products' annual report listed this popular drug's sales as close to half a billion dollars. Its popularity with cardiologists was easy to figure when one knows that heart disease is the world's leading cause of death.

The report made me feel more confident and I decided, excluding an emergency, not to visit my cardiologist till my regular August checkup. At that time, it would be exactly one year since this disturbing change in my life had occurred.

On August 10th I again arrived at my doctor's office and after the regular routine, I finally saw him. It was apparent how busy he was. The waiting room was full. When I finished weighing and stripping to the waist he finally entered the small examination room. When greetings were over and he looked at the folder with my records, it appeared he'd momentarily forgotten he'd received a report from the Cleveland specialist, whom I'd seen for another opinion at the recommendation of Anderson.

He recalled it when I mentioned I'd brought along a copy of the specialist's resume which I'd obtained from a physicians' reference source in our public library. He hurried from the examining room and retrieved his letter. I decided it must have been the first time he'd had time to read it, though later I concluded I might be wrong. When he spoke, I got the impression he wasn't too pleased that the Cleveland doctor's view hadn't supported his own, even though he originally stressed that he always welcomed a second opinion.

Finally we discussed my current medication. He inquired if I wanted to change. I said yes, I'd like to, since the other doctor implied a beta-blocker might help prevent more episodes.

After giving me another EKG and finding nothing that warranted otherwise, he wrote out a new prescription, to be taken once a day, for 50 mg of the beta-blocker, Toprol®. I was to discontinue Isoptin®, the calcium-channel blocker.

I had been on the new drug less than a week, when suddenly, over an eight day period, three new flutter events overwhelmed me. Each one lasted between seven and ten hours. If there were any redeeming qualities to these psychologically debilitating episodes, I was much relieved I'd not developed a stroke. To say the least, I'm sure multiple episodes leave an indelible mark on anyone's brain who suffers from atrial flutter—-life threatening or not. It did on mine. The experiences were physically and mentally most taxing.

Nevertheless, I restrained myself from excitedly phoning the Doc. I didn't want to become a total bore. The word "nuisance" had been used several times by all three cardiologists while explaining *flutter*. The word was ever present in my head. While procrastinating, I also consoled myself by recalling each doctor saying a newly ingested drug often requires more time to "load itself" into one's system. I knew to wait was a gamble on having more episodes, but I decided to wait anyway.

Several weeks passed and the episodes still came and went. While not as frequent, they were still astoundingly very much with me.

After much haranguing to myself, I finally phoned his service. When he returned my call some twenty minutes later and suggested he come to my house, I was grateful.

When he arrived he found me reading in bed where I'd been most of the day. I was feeling more blue than physically impaired.

After listening to my ticker he confirmed it was indeed atrial flutter and suggested I come to his office the next day and "We'll go from there." On his way out, he reminded me it wasn't necessary to remain in bed during these episodes.

I once again concluded he was deliberately reaffirming that this condition was a big, confusing "nuisance," and not "life threatening." These reassuring words were the ones I liked to hear, though they still left me quite baffled.

When he left my home, the arrhythmia was still going on, and I reflected on my visit with the renowned specialist and his suggestion that I change to a beta-blocker. Ironically, I mused on how my own cardiologist, being a normal human being, might find some satisfaction knowing that during the period I was taking his recommended calcium-channel blocker, I'd had only two episodes in a year. Now with the new suggested beta-blocker, I'd recorded three terrifying events in less than a month.

I later learned that these frequent episodes were not unusual when switching from drug to drug. With this malady who's to say who's right. The whole damn thing reminded me of the ancient Chinese water torture that was sinisterly designed to drive one toward insanity one minute at a time. If there was any consolation to all of this, it was my own heart torturing me and not someone else.

The following day's office visit resulted in another EKG and this time, as I expected, it confirmed a perfectly normal and healthy heart. "They're right," I thought. "The cardiologists are right. What a damn nuisance."

After the exam, he suggested I switch immediately from Toprol® to Isoptin®, the trade name for the calcium-channel blocker that had worked so much better for me in the past, though this time he decided I should up the dose of Isoptin® from 180 to 240 mg a day. Though I had read that one should not stop a beta-blocker abruptly, I was confident he knew what he was doing. Maybe, I thought, Isoptin® was close enough to a beta-blocker that it didn't matter. I was much relieved. More mg of Isoptin® was even better, or so I hoped.

Unfortunately, the increased dose of the original drug didn't work as well as it had the first year. I quickly experienced several more arrhythmias over a thirty day period.

Now I was really perplexed and exhausted from

frustration. I speculated the medical profession must be doing a lot of guessing about what to do for arrhythmias. It appeared that atrial flutter was one of those special heart problems they don't quite have a handle on.

IV

INTERACTIVE FOODS

To further my overall confusion I'd recently read an article written by Abigail Zuger in the *New York Times* science section titled, *"How Grapefruit Juice Makes Some Pills More Powerful."* Typical of Zuger and other *Times* writers, she'd done a very thorough job of research and I'd learned as a longtime reader of that section that one could always rely on the accuracy of their stories.

The subtitle of this story carried on to report, "Effect on an enzyme leaves more of some drugs in intestine." Further into the piece Zuger continued, "Researchers have known since 1989 that when some of the common blood-pressure pills called calcium-channel blockers were washed down with grapefruit juice, far more of the drugs reached the blood than when they were taken with a swallow of water, but it is a piece of information that has passed many doctors and patients by, even though the interaction has now been reproduced for other drugs. The effect may be so striking that some scientists are calling for warning labels about the effects of grapefruit juice on pill bottles to prevent drug overdose."

Dr. Paul B. Watkins, a professor of medicine at the University of Michigan in Ann Arbor, whose research recently clarified why grapefruit alone among citrus fruits appears to make some pills more powerful, said, "We are harnessing the power of grapefruit. In some cases an unaccustomed glass of juice in the morning may send enzyme levels plummeting and drug levels soaring as much as ninefold."

The story went on to quote another prominent researcher, Dr. J. David Spence at the Roberts Research Institute in London, Ontario, who thinks this is what may have happened to a Michigan man who died in 1993 with toxic blood levels of Seldane® after drinking two glasses of grapefruit juice. "The issue is that juice is taken intermittently," he said, "And grocers don't take a drug history when they sell it." As I read this tidbit, I'm sure my blood pressure jumped to unreasonable heights.

Quite naturally my grocer, I thought, has never inquired about my drug history, nor for that matter had my doctor inquired about interactive foods, though I truly suppose one can't expect doctors to think of everything regarding each and every patient when they're seeing so many other patients each day. How can they have much time to dwell on me?

My particular concern was in my quest to lose weight. I'd been devouring half a grapefruit a day, (equal to a small glass of juice) while also curtailing my volume of food. Miraculously, with this regimen and other mental gyrations, I'd lost forty-eight pounds within a two year stretch.

Unfortunately for me, it was during that period I experienced some strange side effects. (Headaches, constipation, pains in the kidney area, drowsiness, blurred vision with dizziness.) I now can't help but wonder if it was the interactive grapefruit that was causing them. For my arrhythmias I was simultaneously taking Isoptin®, a calcium-channel blocker.

Near the end of the article Dr. Watkins somewhat reassured the readers, "These are generally safe drugs. I tell my patients if you're used to taking your medication with juice, keep doing it. If you're not, don't start."

More recently (mid-1999) the American College of Clinical Pharmacology notified its membership that Janssen Pharmaceuticals had sent out a letter to health professionals warning them of adverse reactions between grapefruit and the drug, Propulsid® (cisapride).

This is just another indication that wolfing down all kinds of combinations of foods and drugs can have unsuspecting and disastrous effects. If the opportunity presents itself, I firmly believe that those people taking prescription drugs should inquire with their doctors or, at the very least, their pharmacists about grapefruit and the drugs they are taking.

I suspect that more of these notices concerning other types of food and drug combinations will be showing up in the press in the future.

Shortly after that story I ran across another in the Doctors' World section of the *Times* written by Lawrence K. Altman, M. D. It truly didn't help my psyche.

He wrote about another unfortunate drug combination that proved fatal, a combination of a beta-blocker and phenylephrine, sold over-the-counter as Neo-Synephrine® which is used to relieve nasal congestion. In the same article he quoted Dr. Barbara A. DeBuono, then New York State Health Commissioner, as saying, "Even a 'safe' over-the-counter drug can be lethal. Sometimes we take over-the-counter drugs a little less seriously than we would a prescription drug. And overlook the serious side effects."

I began realizing, without much consolation, that both foods and drugs in the wrong combination can be an invitation to the Devil's ball.

One part of Dr. Altman's story that really got my attention was, and I quote, "Doctors are legally free to use a marketed drug for any purpose that they believe is justified." That was indeed, as the cliché goes, a wake up call.

For the first time I consciously realized that my life is truly in the hands of the cardiologists I choose to treat me. If things worked out, fine. If they didn't, too bad for me. At this time I believe there's little chance the doctors will suffer any real consequences.

As much as I love grapefruit, I gave it up and confess I began feeling much better. Then I wondered how many more commonly eaten foods and drugs did not mix well. After mulling over this astounding thought, I reinforced my decision to learn more about how the combination of the two actually affected my medical condition.

V

MORE SIDE EFFECTS

A few weeks later I visited my cardiologist and reported that I'd had several more episodes. Again he decided to change the medication. This time he prescribed Rythmol® (propafenone), 300 mg twice a day. Relatively speaking it was a newly developed drug. I gleaned that information from the library's latest *Physicians' Desk Reference* book. It covers all ethical prescription and over-the-counter drugs.

Rythmol® had not as yet been approved for atrial flutter, though the package insert that came with the prescription did say it was used for sustained ventricular tachycardia, a much more serious heart condition. (The Food and Drug Administration requires all drug manufacturers to incorporate with each package an insert that explains the pros and cons of the drug.) Unfortunately, most people find these inserts impossible to read without the help of a super magnifying glass and superior medical knowledge.

As an aside, in Ellen Goodman's syndicated column of July 2, 1999, she relates that "In 17th Century England there was actually a law that fined a physician if he told a patient what was in a medicine. In 20th Century America, for that matter, there was a government regulation that said drug information had to be written in a language that was unintelligible to the average person."

For my part, in spite of my associations with the drug industry and my constant exposure to technical words, I've decided that things have changed little since the period Goodman was talking about.

The Rythmol® insert made me feel very uncomfortable. It pointed out that this drug was "indicated for the treatment of documented ventricular arrhythmia such as sustained ventricular tachycardia that in the judgment of the physician is life threatening. Because of the proarrhythmic effects of propafenone HCI (Rythmol®), it should be reserved for patients in whom, in the opinion of the physician, the benefits of treatment outweighs the risk. The use of propafenone HCI is not recommended in patients with less severe ventricular arrhythmia, even if the patients are symptomatic."

I was not particularly symptomatic and I didn't have ventricular arrhythmia and could not help but ask myself why the doctor had me on such a strong drug.

Once again I deferred to his judgment. The insert continued to point out that "the use of propafenone HCl for the treatment of sustained ventricular tachycardia, like other antiarrhythmics, should be initiated in the hospital." The doctor had not sent me to the hospital before administering this drug, though I concluded he hadn't because my arrhythmia was much less severe.

Adding to my latest puzzle, the package insert went on to say that "the effects of propafenone HCl in patients with recent myocardial infarction and in patients with supra-ventricular tachycardia have not been adequately studied as in the case of other arrhythmic agents," and it continued, "There is no evidence from controlled trials that the use of propafenone HCl favorably affects survival or the incidence of sudden death." Fortunately for me, I thought, I have neither of these two diseases.

My question to myself was, "Why in the devil am I taking it?" It seemed to me that it was more likely to kill me than cure me.

A short time later, and after the fact, I happily learned the drug was currently with the FDA for approval for the additional indication of atrial fibrillation, though I definitely wondered why, after all those earlier terrible warnings.

Again this left me more confused about my treatment. I wondered why I was getting an atrial fibrillation drug when my cardiologist had clearly diagnosed me with atrial flutter, though I believed he was as up to date about medications as the rest of them.

Unfortunately, it wasn't long before a strange episode appeared and at a most inconvenient time. I had arrived late at night for a few days visit with my young granddaughter in Ocean City, Maryland. It was about an eight hour drive from the Adirondacks. I awakened about six the next morning with my heart clocking 150 beats a minute from a normal 75. I decided I must leave immediately for home to have the episode recorded at my doctor's office on an EKG machine since he'd requested it earlier. Unfortunately, I only had time to say hello and good by to her.

Just as I arrived at his parking lot the episode abruptly stopped. For the first time during one of these damn things I was madder-n-hell it had ceased. It reminded me of the many times I'd taken my car to the dealer for an annoying rattle. As usual, at that particular time the mechanic could never find where it originated.

The following day my doctor called me at home and suggested I increase my dose of Rythmol® another 110 mg to a total of 625 mg a day, and along with it I should take 50 mg of Toprol®. We both hoped the two drugs together would control what, I believed, was my new malady of drug induced *tachycardia*. Tachycardia was another new medical word which I'd learned means a very fast heart rate.

It seemed to be widely published that drug combinations were quite common in treating atrial fibrillation.

Dr. Bramah Singh of the VA Medical Center of West Los Angeles and his colleagues reported in *The Journal of the American College of Cardiology* that, "When the drug digoxin is combined with a beta-blocker, more effective control of heart rate results." It went on to say that "digoxin is the first line therapy for controlling the heart rate in patients with atrial fibrillation, a condition in which the upper chambers of the heart contract, or quiver, ineffectually. If not controlled, atrial fibrillation can lead to serious complications, including stroke.

"The researchers tested 5 different drug regimens in 12 patients with this condition. The treatments included: digoxin alone; a beta-blocker, atenolol; a calcium-channel blocker, diltiazem; digoxin and atenolol; and digoxin and diltiazem. Each patient was treated with each of the 5 different regimens for two-week periods.

"Of all the regimens tested in the same cohort of patients, (digoxin) was one of the least effective agents, both during ordinary daily activities and during treadmill exercise," the investigators wrote. "The best control that we achieved with a single drug was with the beta-blocker. But when we combined it with digoxin, we achieved almost ideal control of the heart rate."

I could only hope that Rythmol® and the beta-blocker, Toprol®, would achieve like results in me even though digoxin and Rythmol® were different types of drugs.

For the next four months, with the change in the drugs to this new regimen, I thought I had hit a home run. I hadn't had an episode and was enjoying a vacation away from my crazy heart.

Suddenly it all changed. I was having my annual physical examination by my internist and learned that I had developed a case of anemia (a condition where the number of red blood cells or the amount of hemoglobin in them is abnormally low, which creates a shortage of oxygen in the blood.)

The internist conferred with my cardiologist and decided that the cause was most likely Rythmol®. The cardiologist said that the package insert also warned of this possible adverse reaction in some patients. As a result of their conference my cardiologist instructed me to discontinue using Rythmol®, continue Toprol® temporarily and start taking 40 mg of Betapace® (Sotolol) three times a day.

A week later I was taken off Toprol® altogether at which time he increased the Betapace® to two 80 mg pills a day. In checking this out, I found that Betapace® works with a dual action. It is both an antiarrhythmic and beta-blocking drug.

Try as I would, I just couldn't overcome that guinea pig feeling. Once again I decided I must expand my research on alternative treatments. This time I vowed I'd follow through all the way. With sound, well informed knowledge I felt certain I could eventually take more control of my own health.

VI

FDA APPROVES QUESTIONABLE DRUGS

Currently I am aware of only three procedures for treating my malady: a drug regimen, radiofrequency ablation, and the maze procedure which requires open heart surgery.

I'm presently on drugs, and from my point of view, too many kinds, combinations and side effects. Also, it didn't help my psyche when I read of all the problems with current FDA approved drugs. As an example, the *New York Times* carried a story by Cheryl Gay Stolberg, "Heart Drug Withdrawn as Evidence Shows It Could Be Lethal. In a rare move, the FDA reverses a decision." The rather detailed story went on to say that the drug, "Posicor®, a calcium-channel-blocker, inhibits certain liver enzymes that enable the body to eliminate other drugs. When the enzyme is not working, the other drugs can build to toxic levels."

Stolberg quoted Dr. Murray M. Lumpkin, deputy director of the Center for Drug Evaluation and Research at the FDA, as saying, "It was too complicated to try to use a drug in the elderly population (I'm almost one of those) when you have more than twenty-five different drugs that you can't use it with." As I read this, I nervously recalled my experience with a calcium-channel blocker and grapefruit and with propafenone HCl (Rythmol®).

The story carried on to point out what most of us already know. That is, that the agency is currently under intense pressure from Congressional Republicans, and I believe Democrats alike (lobbyist money doesn't discriminate), to speed up its drug approval process; it has recently given its approval to 92 new drugs - a record number. Surely these approvals will make the drug companies richer.

As a footnote, I've read of five of these drugs withdrawn from the market because of the unacceptable numbers of deaths.

Ms. Stolberg's story further pointed out that in February '97 "an independent panel of expert scientists voted 5 to 3 to advise the FDA to approve Posicor®. Among those who voted against approval was Dr. Lemuel Moye, a biostatistician at the University of Texas Health Science Center in Houston. Dr. Moye said he was troubled by preliminary data from an ongoing study of 2,600 patients that suggested Posicor® might cause unusual electrical activity in the heart (that's what I'm trying to get rid of). Dr. Moye continued, "I just could not justify voting for this drug in the presence of a finding which may be a harbinger of danger."

To add insult to injury, in November of '98, Rita Rubin wrote a story in USA TODAY, titled, "Staffers say FDA Approves Some Drugs It Shouldn't."

Ms. Rubin was covering the results of a survey that was released by The Public Citizen Health Research Group. "It appears that more than 10% of the FDA's staff who review new drug applications feel that drugs were approved in the last three years that *should not* have been." The consumer advocacy organization had mailed a survey to 172 medical officers involved in such reviews at the FDA. Peter Lurie, who directed the survey, says, "The level of dissatisfaction among the FDA medical reviewers could be even higher, given that about two-thirds did not respond to the survey." The following were some of his findings:

"(1) Nineteen respondents said they felt that a total of 27 drugs they'd reviewed since 1995 received FDA approval when they shouldn't have.

"(2) Nineteen said pressure to approve more of the drugs they review was "somewhat greater" or "much greater" than before 1995.

"(3) Seventeen described the current FDA drug review standards as "lower" or "much lower"; thirteen described them as "about the same", and six described them as "higher."

"The levels of discomfort, the levels of medical officers being overruled, are beyond what we had expected and very worrying from a public health point of view," says Lurie, whose organization has accused the FDA of approving drugs too quickly.

Janet Woodcock, director of the FDA's Center for Drug Evaluation and Research, says, "The public should rest assured that FDA maintains the highest standards in the world for approving drugs." In my opinion this is a typical bureaucratic response.

This story reconfirmed for me that the potential for sloppiness and indifference can always exist in large government bureaucracies.

A few years ago, in my work as a consultant, I had some experience with the FDA and compared to that time I believe their procedures have changed as they are approving drugs faster. I only hope for the sake of patients who depend on these drugs that this doesn't mean they're indeed relaxing their standards.

The March 28, 1999 edition of the *Times* in a front page story by Robert Pear reported that the Federal Government (FDA) has repeatedly reprimanded national drug companies. They are being chastised for making false and misleading claims in television commercials and magazine advertisements covering numerous prescription drugs. Anyone who watches even a smidgen of TV could not help but be saturated with the drug companies' voluminous miracle cures.

In 1998 the FDA singled out many companies about commercials advertising prescription drugs for anything from high cholesterol to high blood pressure, hair loss and sexual diseases. They also raised Cain about birth control pills, weight loss pills, anticancer drugs, and stop smoking regimens. The regulatory agency said their advertisements violated the Federal Food, Drug and Cosmetic Act because they overstated the benefits of a particular drug, minimized the risk or falsely suggested that one drug was superior to another. Likewise, the agency found that drug companies were promoting drugs for other uses not approved by the government.

All the recent advertising aimed directly at consumers stems from a 1997 change in the FDA rules and it appears now that the FDA is having trouble controlling the drug companies much to the detriment of patients.

Dr. David Kessler, former head of the FDA and presently head of the Yale Medical School, asks, "Is it in the public interest to advertise a weight-loss drug which is a controlled substance that can produce dependency?" and "Is it in the public interest to make a mediocre drug the drug of choice based on marketing and not science?"

All this is a clear indication that if the patient isn't very careful, one could become the unsuspecting victim of drug company research doctors who operate under the cloak of the Hippocratic oath. By all that's holy they should be objecting to inappropriate claims by the companies' marketing departments.

Should one need other examples, read Stephen Fried's book, *"Bitter Pills: Inside the Hazardous World of Legal Drugs"* (Bantam). If this one doesn't scare your mule, nothing will.

For starters, Mr. Fried points out that a commentary in the *Journal of the American Medical Association* argued that "vital safety monitoring tasks" were being "largely neglected" and how a more recent *"JAMA (Journal of the American Medical Association)* study and editorial pronounced that more than 100,000 Americans die each year from adverse reactions to prescription drugs, making drug reactions the fourth leading cause of death in the country."

In a more recent study, the not-for-profit Advisory Council to Improve Outcomes Nationwide in Heart Failure published new treatment recommendations in the January, 1999 issue of the *American Journal of Cardiology*. It hopes to bring doctors up to date and encourage them to become more aggressive in applying the new findings. They cited how no more than "5% of the five million Americans with heart failure are receiving the most effective therapy." A panel of 150 cardiologists again estimates 100,000 more deaths annually than otherwise occur.

Following these reports there was another disheartening story in the *Wall Street Journal*. Ron Winslow, one of the staff writers who contributes regularly to the Health page, reported on a new story that had recently appeared in the *Journal of the American Medical Association*. His article, "Heart Researchers Find Beta-Blockers Of Little Benefit in Improving Survival," went on to say that, "Heart researchers reported that a class of drugs widely used to treat high blood pressure provide little benefit when it comes to improving survival or preventing heart attacks among elderly patients."

The WSJ story continued with what I already suspected. "The drugs, known as beta-blockers, have been on the market for about 30 years and are taken by more than 11 million Americans, researchers said. The findings suggest they may be overused among elderly patients who haven't suffered any complications from high blood pressure. All told, about six million elderly Americans take beta-blockers." However, the researchers cautioned that people already on the drug should not stop taking it, except under the direction of a doctor.

Franz Messerli, a blood pressure specialist at the Ochsner Clinic, New Orleans, and lead author of the *Journal of the American Medical Association* article, clearly gave the impression that diuretics were the drugs of choice for high blood pressure in the elderly. He said, "Beta-blockers needlessly expose more than six million elderly with hypertension to the cost, inconvenience and side effects of drug treatment without providing any true benefits."

Later I was advised by Dr. John Mullane, who had obtained FDA approval in 1976 for Ayerst Laboratories' beta-blocker, propranolol (Inderal®), to be used to treat high blood pressure, that it was clear back in the mid 80s that beta-blockers were less effective in the older hypertensive patient. However, he believes that beta-blockers such as propranolol are useful in the elderly to prevent second heart attacks. Propranolol lowers blood pressure more in the young than in the elderly. He believes, as does Messerli, that a diuretic could quite possibly be a better first step choice in the elderly than a beta-blocker.

As for me, with the exception of a diuretic, I've been on a variety of prescriptions, propranolol included, off and on over the past three years.

I've taken one pill a day, two pills a day, three pills a day, and often five pills a day. I've taken them one hour before I eat, two hours after I eat, when I get up, when I go to bed. I've worried about overdosing, underdosing or forgetting to dose at all. I often wonder if some of my other pains aren't due to the many drugs I'm eating. Often I feel like saying the hell with all of them .... but I don't. I certainly have no intention of changing my present medication regimen without my own doctor telling me to, but I do intend to continue exploring the other options that might solve my problem as I urge all fellow sufferers to do.

Apparently there is much confusion among all the doctors about what drug works best. This was recently confirmed to me when I discovered that the National Heart, Lung, and Blood Institute had contracted with Midatlantic Cardiovascular Associates of Baltimore, MD to conduct trials on which of eight drugs was the most effective to use for fibrillation. This new clinical study is "Atrial Fibrillation Follow-up Investigation of Rhythm Management (AFFIRM for short)."

My own conclusions are that there is a close similarity between flutter and fibrillation. At times my own heart when monitored by me has produced the Morse Code rhythm ...–...–...–......–.. and at other times it has been more chaotic as though the electrical impulse had shorted to all parts of my heart with no particular rhythm and could be visualized as an erratic circular motion.

The study's boilerplate says, "The AFFIRM study is a randomized evaluation of treatment of atrial fibrillation by 1 of 2 strategies: ventricular rate control and anticoagulation versus rhythm control and anticoagulation."...."AFFIRM will randomize therapy and follow 4300 patients for an average of 3.5 years (minimum 2 years) at 200 sites in the United States and Canada." The medications used are all approved by the FDA.

According to Ms. Mary Michael the atrial fibrillation study will be completed in the spring of 2002.

I, and millions of others, are anxiously awaiting the results of this very necessary study. The urgent need for this study was confirmed by a December 1999 report released by the National Academy of Science, Institute of Medicine, a most exalted source, that the horrifying numbers of 44,000 to 98,000 people die unnecessarily each year due to medical carelessness.

Dr. Lucian Leape, of Harvard, a co-author of the report said, "that's comparable to having three jets filled with passengers crash every two days. If this were the case every airline in the country would be grounded until the reasons were corrected." Dr. Leape went on to say that, "Health care is a decade or more behind other high risk industries in its attention to insuring basic safety."

He said that the number one cause of medical mistakes is not incompetence, but confusion, and went on to recommend the establishment of a center of patient safety within the Department of Health and Human Services to collect and distribute information about medical errors and error prevention systems.

He also recommends (and in my opinion it's unlikely to ever happen under our present lobbying system) that Congress require all health providers to report mistakes which cause serious injury or death, though presently only 20 states have enacted this.

FDA APPROVES QUESTIONABLE DRUGS

I must agree with another outstanding report appearing in the December 6th, 1999 *Newsweek*, by Dr. Jay S. Cohen, titled, "The One Size Dose Does Not Fit All." To me the title says it all. Often times what's good for the goose, isn't good for the gander. Cohen is an assistant clinical professor of the University of California and the author of "Make Your Medicine Safe." (Avon Books)

VII

CHANGING
DIRECTIONS

That uncertain and confusing information about drugs was enough to speed up my research into the details of these other alternatives that are currently available to the atrial flutter/fibrillation patient.

I already know I'm not presently emotionally prepared for full scale open heart surgery such as the relatively new maze procedure where a surgeon whacks open the chest to get to the heart, then cuts a maze of lines for the electrical charge to travel on. That leaves only radiofrequency ablation or to stay on my present drug regimen.

Ablation to my ears sounds like the lesser of three evils and a damn sight less complicated than the maze procedure. Nevertheless, all of these procedures filled my weary mind with plenty of apprehension.

Again, I discussed my presumed plight with my wife and brought her up to where I believed I stood. We discussed some of the articles I'd received from our neighbor. I reviewed the one I'd already read from the *Reader's Digest,* titled, *When the Heart Misfires*, by Pamela Patrick Novotny, and carefully read *A Heart Out of Control*, by Jane Harriman, a staff reporter for the *Des Moines Register*. They both offered the names of cardiologists who were experienced with ablation. I quickly decided to take the plunge and picked one of the cardiologists the *Digest* mentioned.

Dr. William Miles, an *electrophysiologist* and specialist in electrical heart problems, was, at this time, on the team of Dr. Douglass Zipes. Dr. Zipes is Director of Research at the Krannert Institute of Cardiology at the Indiana University Medical Center and from the article's presentation was obviously one of the pioneers of the ablation procedure. I had no trouble reaching Dr. Miles. He returned my call as soon as he was finished in the operating room. That got my attention. I had concluded years ago that a successful man takes action and knows the importance of responding to an apprehensive caller. His attention and low key talk was more than welcome. The phone conversation was quick and efficient. In minutes I'd given him all the necessary information for him to set me straight about what was involved. He told me at this time they had an eighty-five to ninety percent success rate, though I'd also learned from previous research that in most treatments of any type of heart problem there was always a caveat covering the possibility of doom. I was surprised when he mentioned money - the cost would be approximately $15,000.

I didn't let my questionable thoughts deter me. He continued explaining how he needed a copy of my latest electrocardiogram before he could make a decision as to whether or not I was a "good candidate for ablation." He strongly emphasized "good." Obviously the implication was that not everyone with arrhythmia was automatically a candidate for his services. He went on to say that after reviewing the EKG thoroughly, he'd get back to me with his opinion. In the meantime he wanted his assistant to speak to me. She'd give me more details about what to expect if and when I became a patient.

Ms. Paddock gave me a brief rundown and concluded by telling me she'd send a more detailed pamphlet. I was glad. I'd much rather have a pamphlet that was written for the layman than try to remember everything she'd been saying on the phone. Two days later I received the brochure. It was indeed clear and well prepared. Also, and fortunately, it had been written for the uninformed layman.

Happily, the booklet explained the technical meaning of *electrophysiology*. I had learned earlier the big word simply meant the study of electrical impulses that make the heart pump. I thought back to my earlier, simplistic conclusions that in most cases the workings of the heart are like the power from a car's electrical alternator that produces the spark for a spark plug. When a plug shorts, the engine runs, but runs rough.

The small pamphlet went on to explain that after entering the hospital, the EP studies, as they were known, (*electrophysiologic*) would allow the cardiologist to diagnose the extent and source of the problem. A good bit of the booklet contained routine information, but for the first time during my investigation it more clearly explained in some detail just what *ablation* therapy was all about.

I learned that the procedure was conducted by the catheterization process. A catheter (one or more pliable and insulated long thin wires) was carefully guided, with the help of an X-ray camera, through one of the veins in an arm, neck or groin till it reaches the heart chamber. When the predetermined source of the arrhythmia is reached, the abnormal tissue can be zapped with a low voltage electrical current or by injecting a chemical. That choice is determined solely by the operating cardiologist. The pamphlet went on to explain that after the procedure, there's a lot of careful monitoring of the results and if all goes well the patient would probably be able to return home in a couple of days.

To read that the possibility of someone probing around in one's heart is unnerving, is no exaggeration.

However, it was good to know that even though much of this relatively new approach was experimental, I felt encouraged that medical science had advanced far enough over the last few years to perform this "miracle of medical science."

Certainly, one must have atrial flutter/fibrillation to appreciate the full extent of the frustration one has when the heart is out of control and resulting stroke may be imminent. Often, during a twelve hour episode, I morbidly compared it to being on death row without a defined date and time for my execution. Multiply that by several times over a six month period and it's quite easy to see the impact it can make on one's life.

After some very heavy thinking, I decided to send the EKGs of my first recorded episode of atrial flutter to Dr. Miles and wait impatiently till I heard from him.

A week or so later he called and said that I "might not" be a good candidate for ablation therapy. He startled me when he said, "I don't think you have *atrial flutter*. It appears to me you have *atrial fibrillation*. Unless there was static on the EKG machine when you had this event, I believe it's *fibrillation*. At the moment we're not doing ablation for atrial fibrillation. We may in the future but not now. Nevertheless, the next time you have an episode go immediately to the hospital and record the event on an EKG machine, then forward me the results."

At the time I wondered how the experts formed their conclusions that I had flutter. I was glad to know that the drug therapy for atrial flutter, atrial fibrillation, and tachycardia had major similarities. My esteemed sources said drugs such as beta-blockers, calcium-channel antagonists, Rythmol®, digitalis and many others might be tried by various physicians to suppress or eliminate the occurrence of these damn nuisances.

I spent the next several hours going over and over what Dr. Miles had told me. I then reviewed all the past criteria concerning my condition. I was very unhappy believing I'd been under the wrong impressions. Or had I? Had all the doctors misread my original EKGs, thereby misdiagnosing my arrhythmia, or was Dr. Miles reading the EKGs wrong, I asked myself? Who was right? Could my heart be switching from flutter to fib? If it was, I'd have to forget ablation, stay on drugs or consider the maze procedure.

My inclination was to phone my own doctor and put everything on the line, though I hadn't alerted him that I'd sent the original EKGs to Miles. I hadn't even informed him that I was thinking about having an ablation. I finally concluded that the next time an event took place I'd have his office record it and confirm his original diagnosis of atrial flutter for Dr. Miles.

Fortunately, and I say that reluctantly, I had another episode about a week later. In my doctor's absence another associate performed a brief EKG. He not only confirmed it was indeed atrial fibrillation, he also casually commented that he'd experienced two episodes himself.

For reasons unknown to me, I was damn glad to hear that this cardiologist had also experienced this type of arrhythmia. I felt he really knew what the hell they're all about. When he explained the circumstances about how and when his came, I could sense there was a commonality among the four million or more of us who suffered the same mysterious and little understood plight.

A few days later when I again returned to my own doctor, he made arrangements for me to have another, sophisticated 30 day Event Monitor. This device is much like the Holter Monitor, though this gadget was just slightly larger than a pack of cigarettes, portable, with no wires attached to the body. The nurse explained that during an episode one must press it firmly against the chest and over the heart muscle to record the event. In approximately one minute it completes a recording. The patient is then instructed to call a special 800 number, press the telephone mouth piece to the gadget, push a replay button and a computer at the other end re-records what's happening to the heart. In turn, the company analyzes the information and sends the results of their analysis to the cardiologist.

As bad luck would have it, 10 days later my heart went on the fritz again. I was prepared with the monitor and learned several days later the computer results verified my pump was again out of sinus rhythm and in atrial fibrillation.

Now, I'd become much more discouraged and concluded that when and if they perform ablations on atrial fibrillation patients, I would most likely agree to have it done.

I was particularly encouraged after reading the following e-mail from a survey I conducted. It represents many others expressing their satisfaction with the procedure.

"I had an ablation procedure one year ago to correct Wolfe Parkinson White. I endured symptoms since I was 12 years old and they progressively got worse. I complained to my doctor of rapid heart beats and chest pain for nearly 13 years, and, after many tests and my demand he finally agreed to send me to a cardiologist who immediately recognized the symptoms. I encourage anyone who thinks there is something wrong with their heart to keep going to doctors until something is done. I felt that my doctor didn't believe me since tests did not show a problem. Holter monitors don't always catch the irregular beats since they are only worn for 24-48 hours.

"Ask for an event monitor (much smaller). They can be worn for up to 2 weeks and activated when you are experiencing an episode. My WPW (Wolfe Parkinson White) was so bad (up to 275 beats/min.) that I was given an ablation 2 weeks after it was found. Yes

it is a scary procedure (but painless). An electrophysiol-ogist performed mine and I have been symptom free for an entire year. I am an extremely active person and life is so much better knowing I won't have any more attacks. I encourage anyone with symptoms to get checked out and to those of you who are diagnosed to look into having an abla-tion. The benefits far outweigh the risks."
Signed: Kristene (June 30, 1999)

However, I must add that my research did turn up a few people who indicated they were still having episodes after the ablation procedure. This relatively new approach seemed at the time to be the final bastion for the physically and psychologically downtrodden *flutter* patient. Just recently I was very encouraged to see an editorial in *Circulation*, the publication of the American Heart Association, titled, "Catheter Ablation of Cardiac Arrhythmias. Usually Cure, but Complications may Occur."

They were commenting on a study that covered the history of 1,050 patients in 18 hospitals who underwent this procedure. The arrhythmia ceased in about 95% of the patients, though there were still a few complications and 3 deaths. Apparently the risk of death rises among patients with more serious underlying heart disease. The researchers said there was a 1% risk that patients would eventually need a pacemaker. With the current improvement of these pace-maker devices, ablation seemed like an excellent alternative to drug therapy that I'd be more willing to gamble on.

VIII

STRESS

THAT ELUSIVE EVIL

S ince this whole business of atrial flutter/fibrillation began over three years ago, I'd religiously carried out the doctor's instructions. I'd also carefully read all the packaged inserts that came with the medications and taken my pills within minutes of the recommended times.

In the past I'd been a typical, old-fashioned American gourmand, weighing 248 pounds at a height of 6'1", though I was told many times by doctors that I had heavy bones. Nevertheless, with my new motivation, I'd gradually lost nearly fifty pounds, briskly walked a mile three times a day, gave up my two daily bourbons, replaced my three or four cups of caffeine coffee with that disgustingly bad, decaffeinated stuff. I also sacrificed what little chocolate I'd occasionally enjoyed.

During the onslaught of a cold, I suffered the cough rather than consume the Robitussin. There was no need to give up smoking, since I had never smoked. According to the doctors, all of these desires were taboos for the atrial fibrillation patient.

I'd actually been depriving myself of all my great little vices.....for truly I was in no hurry to discover what was under the grass. In spite of all my efforts, there was still no end to my episodes.

Last, but in no way least, I've tried especially hard to get rid of whatever could be interpreted as that elusive and popular malady called *stress*. It's quite easy to come across the word in every medical journal. It seems to be responsible for most complicated and undiagnosed diseases in the medical dictionary. For over a decade now this topic also seems to crop up in about every credible publication in the nation.

In the June 14, 1999 issue of *Newsweek*, the cover story was "Stress". It carried a picture of an electrified image with strange circular motions emanating from the caricature of a human body. Its subtitles were, "How It Attacks Your Body" and "Fighting Back: What You Can Do".

Jerry Adler's most interesting story, "How Stress Attacks You," was as conclusive about stress's effects as anything I've read to date. He points out that, "Stress isn't just a catchall complaint; it's being linked to heart disease, immune deficiency and memory loss. We're learning that men and women process stress differently and that childhood stress can lead to adult health problems. The worst part is, we inflict it on ourselves." His charts were most convincing on how this malady plays a role in our unhealthy lives. And while I have little doubt that most everything he points out is true, I'm firmly convinced that the best way that I can protect myself from stress is to become a monk somewhere in Tibet and forget that the real world exists.

Until I read this and a report by Susan J. Wells in the *New York Times*, I often thought the effects of stress on the mind and body were somewhat exaggerated.

Ms. Wells reported in a recent story titled "Deadlines, Dismissals and Health," subtitled, "Heart Risk Tied to Job Situation," clearly seemed to confirmed what Adler and many others already believed.

"Being a manager is tough work. Now it turns out, it may pose a serious and deadly health risk, too. Managers run twice the normal risk of a heart attack the week after they dismiss an employee or face a high-pressure deadline, according to a medical study published last month in the journal *Circulation*." Cynically, it could be interpreted as pay back time.

"Researchers interviewed almost 800 hospital patients between 1989 and 1994 who were employed at the time of their heart attacks—asking them specifically about the occurrence of four job related events; working under a high-pressure deadline; having to dismiss someone; getting a promotion or a raise, and quitting or being laid off.

"Two situations came up as producing the strongest risk of heart attack - having to fire someone and working under a high-pressure deadline," said Dr. Murray Mittleman, an author of the study and a general internist at the Beth Israel Deaconess Medical Center at Harvard University.

The Center for Corporate Health at Beth Israel Deaconess, "estimates that 60 to 90 percent of all medical office visits in the United States are for stress-related disorders and that as much as 80 percent of all disease and illness is initiated or aggravated by stress.

"But this latest study," Dr. Mittleman said, "is the first to focus on and link specific, brief events at work to heart attacks that can occur as many as seven days later."

"So much of our work mentality is warlike combat, us against them," said Joseph Loizzo, a psychiatrist and director of the Center for Meditation and Healing at the Columbia-Presbyterian Medical Center in New York.

The *Times* piece carried on with a story about Patricia Chapman, 55, who was an investment professional at a Fortune 100 high-technology company in Silicon Valley and how she knows first hand the ill effects of stress. Her physician diagnosed her with cardiac arrhythmia in 1989, and she was forced to take a four-month medical leave of absence in 1995 after her condition was aggravated by the pressure of increased job responsibilities and a divorce. Doctors had told her she was at risk for sudden death, her heart was logging 700 extra beats an hour. "Stress was literally killing me," she said. "I was really afraid I was going to drop dead at work."

After years of medication and multiple surgeries offered mixed success, Ms. Chapman took a new approach—a series of techniques taught by Heart Math, a training and consulting company in Boulder Creek, California.

The idea is to quietly use positive thoughts to physically alter and calm the heart's rhythm during stress—in effect, telling the brain to decrease the number of beats. Ms. Chapman, for example thinks for several minutes of a person she loves or of a sports activity she enjoys.

Heart Math said these visualization techniques have been used in employee training programs at Motorola, Shell and Hewlett-Packard.

Many experts note, however, that on-the-job stress remains pervasive.

"The truth is," said Dr. Mittleman of Beth Israel, "we don't know whether certain stress-management practices really will make a difference in reducing death and disability from heart disease."

Subsequently, there appeared an article in my local newspaper, the Glens Falls, NY, *Post Star*, Health and Science section, an article they reprinted from the Fort Worth *Star-Telegram*, titled, "Beware the Hostile Heart." Dr. Redford Williams, who is affiliated with Duke University Behavioral Medicine Research Center, has been warning for years that cynicism is part and parcel of a hostile personality and that a hostile personality can kill us. Now Williams has come up with a short self-test published in the August issue of *Consumer Reports* on health, to determine whether we are too hostile for our own good. They spanned the gamut of angry emotions exercised in our daily lives. The paper said that most researchers believe that the more often we get angry, the greater our risk of heart attack, no matter how we handle that anger.

Apparently, they believe that anger can kill by speeding up the heart rate and making blood pressure soar in such a way that the deposits on coronary arteries are disrupted or clots are formed. It can also narrow the coronary arteries just when the heart muscle needs extra blood and even inhibit certain signals that help maintain normal heart rhythm.

By the time I finished reading these accountings I was closely analyzing myself to determine if there were indeed some stress areas in my life I was foolishly overlooking. At the time I couldn't think of a thing. After all, I'd had 45 years of running my own international consulting firm in New York City, the world's greatest high pressure city. I was now retired with a comfortable income. My wonderful wife of 41 years was healthy and of our four children, three were happily married and living healthy and productive lives, the fourth, still single and contented. My granddaughter was growing into a lovely young lady and I'm pleased about the recent birth of our grandson.

Our home was most comfortable and pleasant. We traveled both in this country and Europe whenever the mood struck us. (And when we could get a baby sitter for our dog!) We had owned large boats, small boats, second homes, and a ski and hunting lodge in the Adirondacks. We've recently purchased a winter retreat in Florida. We've enjoyed the pleasures of several close, long term friends, who were quite willing to endure my idiosyncrasies as I was theirs.

So what else was there?...... Could it possibly be the reams of information I'm hearing and reading on the national media about bad drugs, bad doctors, bad hospitals, questionable HMOs and insurances plans, and unethical politicians to boot? If these books and articles didn't stress me, they probably should have.

When I first experienced atrial flutters (as originally diagnosed), while on the stress test machine, I repeated to myself many times over how I very much wanted to spend a little more time with my grown children and their families to help make up for the many times I was unable to be with them when they were young and I was always traveling. One of my closest friends had often told me that I was a person who enjoyed being in control. I'm sure he was right and now with this damn A-fib thing, I was faced with something it seemed I had no control over at all.

In the past I'd often experienced the uncomfortable feeling of this lack of control when riding in the back of a commercial airliner, and not knowing just how competent the pilot was. Over the years I'd worked hard to adjust myself and to suffer the smaller, more crowded corporate jets because, at the very least, I could be up front with the captain. While measuring his ability to get me safely to my destination, I could also view what was out there in the sky in front of me.

With stress in mind, I once again decided to think more about general health and the doctors' impact on any stress I may have. In 45 years I had had only one other doctor I could actually compare my cardiologist with and the way each of them handled me seemed miles and miles apart.

IX

LEARNING FROM DR. WELBY

My first experience with a civilian doctor after World War II was very gratifying. He was a very successful and prominent general practitioner in New York City. I'd visited him once a year for an annual checkup for over twenty-five years. By today's standards Dr. Craig Smith's approach would be quite novel.

When I first arrived at his office in 1958, I was surprised to see I was the only one in a pleasantly furnished living room like environment. It also appeared my new doctor had no associates in his office.

We sat in the "living room" visiting for twenty minutes. Not once was I asked about my medical history. The conversation seemed more social. It was more about my personal life style, about what I do, where I do it, etc. He showed a genuine interest in my family, their activities in New York City, my children's schools, and where we had lived prior to coming to the big city.

At that time, as a young consultant with employees and offices around the world, I thought he was wasting my valuable time and I wanted to get on with the general examination. Finally he invited me into his inner office and sat me down next to his desk while he queried me on my past medical background. He was taking his questions from a list that covered every subject on health a doctor could dream up.

At the very least it took a half hour to go through them. When his exercise of my memory was over, I was ushered into the examination room, given a robe and asked to strip to my skivvies. He checked me over from the tip of my head to my toes, including all my orifices. At the conclusion of his probing I experienced my first EKG (electrocardiogram). He placed multiple wires all around my heart. They were connected to a small unobtrusive brown box that recorded the heart's actions on a chart. The box reminded me of the barometric pressure instrument in the window of the RCA building at Rockefeller Center where my office was located. As he observed the box's meter he explained all the funny little vertical and horizontal lines that represented the actions of my heart. When the procedure was finished, we returned to his inner office, where once again he went over every detail of his examination and the EKG.

Over the years he would point his pencil to the EKG readout and tell me that I was drinking too much coffee, and I was, and this was precipitating PVCs, "skipped beats" to the layman. He also added that approximately 75 percent of the population "enjoy these abnormalities." At the end of an unhurried hour and twenty minutes he concluded I was in excellent health and didn't, barring some unforeseen development, need to visit him again for at least a year.

As I left his office, I recall thinking about his thoroughness and how lucky I'd been to have found such an excellent doctor. I also more fully understood why he spent the first twenty minutes of social visiting at the very outset.

A year later, on my second visit, I was prepared for a much shorter visit. I was wrong. He covered the same ground he'd covered the year before. When I asked him why he did the repeat, he looked surprised as he asked me, "How in the world could you expect me to remember the answers to all these questions from one year to the next? To me each visit is the same as the first." For the next thirty years till his retirement, he followed the same procedures.

At that time, I suspect most doctors handled patients about the same way. When his bill came I was amazed at how little I was charged for his high quality service. The amount wasn't even close to the hourly rate I was charging companies for our firm's management consultants. Using an educated guess today, the charges for twenty minutes of a typical intimidated and hurried visit to the doctor's office, cost about 900 percent more, which is vastly greater than the wild weed growth of inflation.

X

MAGIC ON THE INTERNET

Fortunately, I had discovered computers as early as 1982. As a long time gadgeteer, I was fascinated with them and spent many extra hours learning all of their revolutionary benefits. Our company used them for all of our accounting as well as establishing a data base for research management information. We also used them for communications between offices, long before e-mail.

By 1993 the whole world had discovered the World Wide Web (www) and the rest of it. It wasn't long before the value of this new research tool became indispensable for me, thousands of other people, and companies alike. The Net grew like wildfire and up sprang a new growth of links (links are Web pages that are linked together by common subjects).

A recent article, "Hospitals Reaching New Patients On Line", written by Lisa Napoli of the *New York Times,* said "As the Internet grows so does the amount of health information available on line, but the sheer volume of information available on the Web does not equal a speedy or accurate search. To give order to the chaos of the Web a handful of healthcare organizations have put their imprimaturs on information-rich Web sites accessible to anyone with a modem."

Ms. Napoli is quite correct. I've already discovered that one should be very selective in searching for information by using the Web sites of hospitals to determine if the medical malady their interested in is a major speciality with these hospitals. I've done this in my quest for information about those who are at the top of the list who deal with atrial fibrillation, radiofrequency ablation, and the maze procedure. Had I not concentrated on the experts in these fields, I could easily have become stuck in a quagmire of confusion.

I hadn't surfed the Net very long before running across the Web site http://www.mediconsult.com. That was indeed a fortunate break. Under Heart Disease I quickly found a link dedicated to *"Atrial Fibrillation."* It answers many good questions for the layman, but it also leaves a lot to be told that can, in my opinion, only be explored with other people who have similar problems. I found a support group on mediconsult.com made up of hundreds of people inquiring about their own health problems and who eagerly exchange information.

I was glad to find the link detailed and user friendly. I quickly discovered the heading, "All You Ever Wanted To Know About *ATRIAL FIBRILLA-TION.*" The subheadings were broken down into the following sections: "Introduction....A Few Fundamentals ....What is *Atrial Fibrillation?*....Who gets *Atrial Fibrillation?*....What are the Symptoms of *Atrial Fibrillation?*....Does Being in *Atrial Fibrillation* Damage my Heart?....What Heart Medication do I need?....What if the Heart Medications Don't Work?....Is *Atrial Fibrillation* a Serious Problem?"

While this information covered a lot, it obviously could not cover everything, though the first time reader can glean enough information to get pointed in the right direction.

In summary, the page seemed to verify most of the doctors' conclusions that if one has an underlying heart disease or chronic atrial fibrillation, it can indeed be more serious. If the arrhythmia is the same as had been diagnosed for me.....*lone, idiopathic, or paroxysmal atrial fibrillation,* the future consequences are not quite as dismal.

The thousands of individuals who've registered with mediconsult.com (it's free) are actively using this site to compare notes and exchange information about their personal medical care. As a huge bonus they can also direct more technical inquiries to a qualified

Mediconsult doctor.

Of course mediconsult.com is not the only health site on the Internet. There's also Mediscape.com, Medline.com, WebMD.com, InteliHealth.com, and I'm sure many others can be reached through one of the many search engines like Yahoo, Excite, Astra Vision, Microsoft's Internet Explorer, AOL, etc.

Equally available are the Web pages of all major hospitals in both this country and abroad. They cover all of their health care activities. To find these hospitals through one of the search engines simply requires typing in the hospital's name, followed by .org. They will then provide the inquiring person with a complete breakdown of all of their services.

For example, in the past the Mayo Clinic provided volumes of written material covering health information and recently started offering CD Roms of health information. It also maintains a Web site (www.mayohealth.org) with a dozen full time editorial workers who publish medical news daily. Each story is reviewed by at least three physicians, according to Dr. Brooks Edwards, its medical editor. The great benefit of Mayo Clinic, Johns Hopkins (www.intelihealth.com) and most all the other major hospitals is that they can provide expert information to multitudes of people who are not in close proximity to their facilities. Mayo's Dr. Edwards said, "In a busy month Mayo Clinic sees 40,000 patients, though a busy month on our Web page brings 1.5 million inquiries."

Making such information available on the Internet and its powerful research machines clearly allows patients the opportunity to arm themselves with knowledge prior to visiting a doctor and it enables them to ask more intelligent questions and in some cases can put their doctors on the spot.

There are many other reasons prompting Internet users to turn to the Web for answers. For example, Michael Stroh of *The Baltimore Sun* in an article, "Unhappy Patients Turn to Online Doctors," wrote about a half dozen physicians glued to computers and making virtual house calls to people they have never heard of and, obviously, will never see. One of the Web sites is America's Doctor, which receives 500,000 hits a month. These new groups are changing the face of American medicine. They offer physicians who answer medical questions directly and – in some cases – even diagnose patients and issue prescriptions. Thousands of medical consumers, frustrated by the assembly pace of managed care are turning to America's Doctor (www.americasdoctor.com) as well as sites such as CyberDocs (www.cyberdocs.com "Where the Doctor is Always In") and WebMD (www.webMd.com "Pay an Office Visit to the Future of Health Care.")

Dr. David Stern, an assistant professor at the University of Michigan Medical School, said, "People are saying, 'I want my doctor to spend more time with me.'" and he added, "I think they are not getting the attention they need, they want, they deserve."

I mostly agree with Dr. Tom Ferguson who is editor of the Ferguson Report in Austin, Texas. His publication monitors online health care industries. "The role of the patient is shifting from someone who just passively follows doctor's orders to people who are taking charge of their own health care."

I feel that anyone suffering from any disease should follow their doctor's advice, but I also firmly believe that each time a patient visits a doctor, they should prepare a list of questions briefly written stressing their concerns about their drugs and his advice. In the end this new Internet revolution will benefit the entire population.

It is interesting to note that until recently doctors were not regarded as one of the groups using this technology for patient communication, though now according to a recent survey of 10,000 doctors, Healtheon Corporation, found that 85 percent are now using the Internet and they pointed out that this is an 875 percent increase from 1997.

Dr. David Voran, a family practitioner in Kansas City, Kansas, regularly keeps in contact by e-mail with many of his patients. "A large amount of what we do really doesn't require an office visit."

It's clear to me that virtual medicine is only going to become more common as the traditional health care industry works harder to adjust to the needs of disgruntled patients.

One should definitely not overlook the Web pages of the leading medical journals, such as the *Journal of the American Heart Association, The New England Journal of Medicine* and myriad others.

As I moused my way through my own support group's link, I was fascinated to read how many of the Web users were experiencing the same apprehensions I'd experienced. One of the postings could easily have been written by me, though older than I am, he writes:

"I am a healthy 73 year. old male. I feel completely well. Today I went to the cardiologist for a routine checkup and was told that I am in atrial fibrillation with a (heart) rate of 120. The M.D. put me on Coumadin and Lanoxin immediately and I am scheduled for a cardiac ultrasound tomorrow. In the meantime I am scared that I will have a stroke any minute. What should I be looking for and should I remain calm with no activity? Please respond ASAP, I am a wreck! Also the doctor mentioned cardioversion if these medications fail."

Signed: Anonymous

This Internet user's desperate sounding e-mail prompted me to gather hundreds of other addresses of those people who were experiencing arrhythmias and send them a detailed questionnaire to solicit their comments for my research.

In a matter of days the answers began appearing on my computer's e-mail site.

Several discussed their experiences with both the ablation and the maze procedures as well as the drugs they were taking. The following selected replies were highly illuminating:

(1)"Having put up with about 3-4 bouts per year of full-blown A-fib over the past twenty years, certain indications of common threads seem to have evolved. A feeling of pressure in the chest (such as gas) prior to an A-fib episode; turning from the waist abruptly and even lying down on my left side, may have triggered these attacks. My doctor does not see any relevance, but my own 'gut' feeling tells me otherwise."

(2)"I, too, have a propensity for A-fib bouts when I lie on my left side, or even when I twist towards the left in a certain way. That's just my perception, but I wish that with all those A-fib sufferers, doctors would look at this more seriously. Maybe what we all need is a doctor with chronic atrial flutter/fibrillation."

(3)" I've been under the care of a cardiologist since 1977. I've had periodic echoes done, and the results were normal. I've also had stress tests with dye and a series of pictures to show blood flow. The results of these tests were also normal. My brother (age 39) has the same condition. In fact, our first A-fib attacks occurred only weeks apart. Apparently there have been recent discoveries of a gene that is responsible for A-fib tendencies (see recent information on subject at end of this e-mail) and in a percentage of cases where it appears to be a family trait. Sunburn always brings on extreme heart irregularities. My gut feeling (no pun intended) is that certain nerves, perhaps the vagus, are too easily set off."

In the March 27, 1997 edition of the *New England Journal of Medicine* there was an extensive article on this subject. It was titled, "Identification of a Genetic Locus for Familial (family history) Atrial Fibrillation." The study was presented by Dr. Ramon Brugada, of the University of Barcelona, et al. His group described three families, all from the same region of northern Spain. "21 of the 49 family members had atrial fibrillation. Two had died of cerebrovascular accidents at 36 and 68 years of age. Of the 19 living family members, 18 had chronic atrial fibrillation, whereas 1 had paroxysmal atrial fibrillation. In none of these patients could a specific cause of atrial fibrillation, such as hypertension, valvular disease, or hyperthyroidism, be found." The study went on to point out that, "Although *familial* atrial fibrillation is extremely rare, the important question raised by this study is to what extent genetic defects may be risk factors for the development of atrial fibrillation. Hypertension, ischemic and rheumatic heart disease, and congestive heart failure are well-known clinical risk factors for atrial fibrillation. On the other hand, no underlying heart disease can be detected in a considerable proportion of patients with atrial fibrillation."

It seems to me that someday we will learn whether other subtle genetic abnormalities are responsible for some cases of lone AF.

(4)"I am unable to wear any clothing that is not entirely without restraint around my mid-section, starting from just under my rib cage, and all the way down. I mean the slightest thing will trigger palpitations. I, too, have been told it is not serious, but it seems to be getting worse. I had the twenty-four hour monitor. I feel the doctors simply do not know. And it is very scary. And yes, overeating can set it off."

(5)"Just recently I went to a cardiologist. Report is 'Live with it and avoid whatever seems to trigger it.' He mentioned that other people have mentioned to him that turning to the left will trigger it. He also said that the upper and lower chambers can decide to work independently. Exercise seems to help, as has losing weight."

(6)"I am 41 years old and had the first episode of A-fib last December. I was very stressed. A few months ago in September I had another episode and a third one a few weeks later. They last about 24 hours. Then the heart goes back to normal, but I don't. I remember the first time it happened. I was urinating a lot. I think this fib is somehow connected to the urination problem (adrenaline), but I don't understand how it works. They say it's an electrical problem, but there is nothing wrong with my heart: the blood pressure is fine; the echocardiogram, too. I'm afraid these medicines I'm taking will have a negative impact on my heart in the long run, but I realize that it is important to take something to keep the heart from going crazy again."

If all this seems confusing to the layman, just think of it from the doctor's point of view. One can now more easily see how they could develop the attitude that atrial flutter/fibrillation is indeed a damn nuisance.

If the cardiologist has fifty atrial flutter/ fibrillation patients visiting him two or three times over the course of year, each with a different story about what brings on the arrhythmia, it seems to me his only recourse is to follow his own personal instincts based on experience and rely on what works best for the majority of his patients. In all probability his treatment of this condition comes from his personal experience, which in some cases I'm sure could be different from that of other cardiologists.

I found the next two e-mails especially interesting, and therefore, I'm including them in their entirety so the reader can get an idea of the types of survey responses the rest of the quotes came from.

(7)"Sit back and get yourself a cup of tea (herbal), this is going to take a while. I am not by nature a hypochondriac but this condition interests me, particularly since it has taken 50% of the wind out of my sails.

"For a number of years, I have had intermittent

episodes of AF, lasting from a few minutes to a half an hour. Then, after a year of extremely high anxiety work, I was hit with a big one (or so I thought at the time). The local hospital ICU had a vacancy so they obliged by taking me and my money for a night. No big deal, but they tried to make the most of it. After that, AF became more and more prevalent. Off to the doctor(s) I went. Each one cautiously agreed with the results of the EKG machine which printed out, the words, "Atrial Fibrillation." "Here, eat these pills!" they would say. First we tried good old Digoxin, .25mg along with Disopyramide Phosphate 150. Nothing! We tried all sorts of beta-blockers. Still nothing.

"Finally, I went to the USA to see Dr. Marc Platte at the Loma Linda Heart Center. Dr. Marc is a specialist in the teeny-weenie area of electrocardiology. He took one look at me and said, "You have asympathetic atrial fib, not sympathetic atrial fib!" I felt better already. So, in somewhat the manner of a stand up comic, Dr. Marc proceeded to tell me that there are two kinds of AF, the sympathetic kind and its evil twin brother, asympathetic AF. Well, that solves the whole problem; right?...Wrong. Dr. Platte suggested that I get back on caffeine of all sorts and small amounts of wine (oh, by the way, I had been off all sorts of nasty old caffeine and the hooch for over two and a half years!) Then Dr. Platte prescribed mega-doses of magnesium (SLO-MAG) several times a day. Zip!! No change except that I ate lots of chocolate and drank a lot of wine. Over time, the problem of sustained AF seemed to become so normal that it would have been abnormal if it had stopped.

"A year passes. Shortness of breath, shortness of memory, lack of solid thinking skills and shortness of other things I really don't want to talk about. I did notice one thing, however. If I concentrated reeeeeal hard on a single sentence, I could make the AF stop —- for a while. If I were to say to myself, "This is purely psychosomatic," the bloody things would stop — for a few minutes. This led me to believe that this situation was purely psychosomatic! How's that for a revelation?

"One day, I wandered into the office of Dr. Arcega, a ticker-tuner in Seattle. Ironically, a number of his tests were made during real live AFs. One AF was a real doozer! In one echocardiogram, I hit over 200 beats per minute. I was really rocking. Another, I clocked almost 300!! Dr. Arcega suggested we look at putting in a pacemaker. Well, I really don't like mechanical gizmos running my life, liberty, and pursuit of happiness, so I respectfully declined the good doctor's offer. After a few minutes of thumbing through his pill book, the good doctor handed me a packet of pills and said, "Eat this." So, I did. What do you know, the AFs went away.

"It has been a year with no serious AFs. Unfortunately, the AFs were replaced by some rather strong heart pounding, especially when I lie down. This is particularly true when I have had another high anxiety day. These high anxiety days seem to range about 360 days per year.

"Back to this miracle drug. The name of the medicine is DILTIAZEM HCL (HERBESSER 90 X 2) 180MG per day plus Digoxin .25mg/day. These seem to do the trick. There is a dark side to these two potions. Swelling and discomfort of the hands and especially the feet. However, Dr. Arcega later suggested changing to VERAPAMIL 120 TO 180 MG per day, accompanied by a dose of Digoxin.

"My conclusion in this whole matter is that atrial fibrillation (in my case) is mainly due to an inability to deal with anxiety (note that I did not say stress). Anxiety and stress are two very distinct conditions. I will let you deal with this one.

"Anyhow, so much for my tale of the atrial fibs.

"I hope you can make some sense out of this. I also hope you can cause some doctor-types to get a little more serious about the causes of AF rather than stuffing pills down peoples' throats. Let me know what you find."

Signed: Survey Participant

Another Responder:

(8)"I am a 51 year old female."I had my first attack about around the age of 47. "I have been under an M.D.'s care since the 2nd or 3rd attack. The first attack came after a long day shopping and running in NYC and eating a frozen yogurt on the way home on the train, so even tho' it lasted 12 hours or so, I attributed it to fatigue and sugar consumption and thought it would never happen again. But I think I had had brief attacks before and never paid them any mind. Anyway, about 6 weeks later I had another attack and became more concerned. I think it was the third attack, again at about a 6-week interval that sent me to the emergency room. But by the time they took a cardiogram, I was back in sinus rhythm. I then went to see a cardiologist who sent me home with a monitor to use when I got the next attack. That was again at about a 6-week interval. That time I was able to electronically transmit the results, and was diagnosed with A-fib and immediately put on digoxin.

"Various medications followed. The digoxin was paired with Cardizem® — unpleasant in itself, but the digoxin only made my condition worse. I was still having attacks about every six weeks which lasted about 12 hours. The digoxin was withdrawn, but I stayed on the Cardizem® for a while. Because the results were less than hoped for, I switched to Betapace® and for awhile that worked fairly well except that the frequency of the attacks increased to once every four weeks, then every three and they began lasting longer, sometimes up to 24 hours.

"I was becoming increasingly depressed and feeling defeated. There was discussion about Cordarone® and flecainide but I was afraid of the possible side effects. Eventually I was driven to considering changing medication. In order to test for the appropriateness of taking flecainide, I was sent for a persantine stress test, (treadmill test would not have worked because the Betapace® prevented my heart rate from exceeding 100bpm.) The test was horrific. I felt like I would implode and explode simultaneously. However, the results were good, proving I had no blockages of any sort.

"At about the same time I saw an electrophysiologist, who said he did not believe an ablation would be of any use and who said that I was too young and not in permanent A-fib so a pacemaker was not a feasible solution. He explained that unlike a pacemaker for bradycardia, the AV node would have to be totally ablated and that I would be entirely dependent upon the pacemaker. This made the ablation procedure one of ultimate last resorts.

"He suggested that since the Betapace® was not working (I was now up to attacks every 10 days), that I just go off medication altogether and see what happened. I did and the result was disastrous. I was going in and out of A-fib every other day. My life was totally disrupted. I couldn't work, I worried constantly about how I could possibly go on, I felt horrible and more depressed than I ever had. I had constant thoughts about killing myself.

"When I realized that I was ready to kill myself, I

also realized that I was ready to take a medication that might have dangerous side effects. We had recently moved and the new cardiologist I was seeing was pretty forceful about my trying Cordarone®. One of the doctors in this group practice had been on the medication for 17 years and when I spoke to him he convinced me that I had to try it. He also convinced me that it would not go away by itself and would probably deteriorate into permanent A-fib. Apparently there are people in permanent A-fib who don't even know they have it, but I will never be one of those people. So, out of desperation, I tried it.

"The medication requires a loading period and for me the prescribed 10 days at a higher dosage didn't work so the doctor felt he was not enough of an expert to deal with my case and wanted to send me to someone else. I wanted to hang in there however, because I couldn't deal with yet another doctor. I wanted to believe that he could help me. So I suggested that we continue the higher dose (600mg/day) for another week and I got lucky. It started working.

"I have been on the medication for 1 year now, and have averaged between 7 and 14 weeks between attacks. A far cry from every 10 days. The doctor said I would continue to have breakthroughs but that given the tenacity of my condition and my resistance to other medications, that I was experiencing a pretty substantial improvement. I feel that I have my life back again and think about the future with the conviction that I will not get worse. Of course there is no guarantee, but I see this as buying time until they figure out how to really help us.

"I did notice some interesting relationships before I was on Cordarone® and digestion. I found that if I ate an especially wonderful meal in a really good restaurant, and had a glass of wine, that I was putting myself in jeopardy of an attack. But then I was sitting in a straight chair, fully dressed, etc. Normally, at home, I change into my robe before dinner and I usually sit on the couch when I have dinner and watch TV so I am much more relaxed. Another interesting thing was that I was constantly having these sort of mini-hiccups and that I don't think many attacks began that weren't preceded by one of these. I noticed in the instructions that came with my mother's pacemaker that hiccups could be an indication that the pacemaker might need an adjustment so I mentioned this to two cardiologists who both sort of shrugged. One said that the arrhythmia might be causing the hiccups as well as vice-versa or that there might be no connection at all. But I am sure there is a connection. Especially that since I have been on the Cordarone® this rarely happens.

"Also my chiropractor was at a conference in which the diaphragm was discussed as a possible related factor. I know there is something to it.

"I also read of work being done at Baylor

University on the genetic connection in A-fib and believe they are onto something in a big way since my brother has the same condition and it began for him at the same age as for me. This is the breakthrough I'm hoping will hold an answer and a cure.

"For now I continue to take my 400mg of Cordarone® a day, although the doctor suggested I try cutting it down to 200. I have to have a chest X-ray each year as well as a pulmonary function test, full batteries of blood tests, etc. Cordarone® has quite a list of possible bad side effects but so far I'm okay. Additionally, the Betapace® depressed my hdls which are now back up to 55 while my ldls have dropped me back into a low risk group for coronary heart disease. Also, I might add, I have no enlargement of the heart, which is a good predictor for success with Cordarone®. I also have mitral valve prolapse (borderline—which means some doctors might say yes and some not—which may be a contributing factor.)

"Well, I had no idea I was going to write so much...please let me know where your research leads you."

Signed: Survey Participant.

As a follow-up to this participant's e-mail, I'm injecting her most recent developments as she reported them to me. Though I feel I'm jumping somewhat ahead, I think it's appropriate to enter it here.

(8A)"Last week we went down to Georgetown

University to see Dr. Cox about the maze procedure. Unfortunately, he had to leave early on the day of my appointment so we didn't get to meet him. But we met with his assistant and the nurse who "runs" the program and I left with a tentative appointment to have the surgery on July 22!!!

"I have not been at all well since the winter. I think I wrote you about the nosebleed that landed me in the hospital for 4 days in March. It's been downhill since then, more and more attacks and afraid to take the Coumadin anymore. So when Les ——- wrote me about a young woman he was in correspondence with who was going for the surgery it piqued my interest. If you recall, you were the first one to mention Dr. Cox to me so I was more receptive to getting in touch with her and finding out what was going on.

"She is a very positive young woman of 38 who has been a "fibber" since she was 23. So you can imagine what it meant to her to have a chance at being cured. Well–she had the surgery on May 5 and went home on the 14th. "The amazing maze!" She is absolutely fine and has been in sinus rhythm since the moment they fixed her. Not everyone does that well at first, but the track record, as I believe you know is excellent.

"I was very impressed with what I saw and heard at Georgetown–I think these are probably among the best MD's in the world. So, since the catheter ablation procedure seems to be stuck without good results, this is the only way I can see to get my life going again. Les — is fighting with the Ministry of Health in Australia to get his insurance to pay for the surgery here for him since it is not done (we don't think) in Australia and there are no doctors anywhere with Dr. Cox's experience. The surgery is very expensive–around $60,000–(including hospital and Dr.) so insurance is a real issue. But based on Lisa's experience we are convinced that we will survive the whole thing and end up cured. He is pretty symptomatic too so there really isn't much of another choice. I'm thankful that this exists now for me even if some years down the pike there may be an easier cure. I just don't want to lose any more years.

"In addition, the amiodarone did its dirty work on me. I have been off it for almost 4 weeks now. It totally messed up my thyroid (I'm now hyperthyroid) and so we have to wait until it is functioning normally before they can do the surgery."

Actually I originally recommended that my Internet friend visit Dr. Cox and it seems apparent that's she's pleased with the results. Later on in this work I will be covering Dr. Cox and his maze procedure in far greater detail.

If all these comments aren't confusing enough, I'll add a few more samples of one liners from hundreds of questionnaires of other perplexed souls searching for answers to what's behind the mystery of atrial fibrillation.

(9)"I gave up chocolate and alcohol and have not had an event since."..... "A lot of twisting and middle body movement can bring on an episode."

(10)"The atrial fibrillation occurred while I had a stomach ache."

(11)"I can definitely relate A-fib to after meal experiences. I always feel PVCs (premature ventricular contractions) after eating."

(12)"I don't get any warning before it happens."

(13)"I would go into A-fib by turning on my left side."

(14)"Before taking Solotol strenuous exercise could trigger an episode. Now it never does."

(15)"Abrupt changes in heart rate, i.e., interval training while swimming, quick starts and stops."

(16)"My doctor also suggests heavy snorers (which I am) produces adrenalin at night in order to breathe and this can also cause A-fib."

(17)"I, too, experience the flutters when I lay on my left side, bend over too rapidly or when I'm highly stressed or nervous."

(18)"If I eat cheese I go into A-fib."

(19)"I had A-fib two years ago clearly traceable to a night of heavy drinking."

(20)"My feeling of pressure in the chest (such as gas) prior to an A-fib episode."

(21)"I, too, have a propensity for A-fib bouts when I lay down on my left."

(22)"Apparently there has been a recent discovery of a gene that is responsible."

(23)"The act of drinking fluid, particularly cold, also brings on fluttering and sometimes full blown A-fib."

(24)"I attribute it to fatigue and sugar consumption."

(25)"I'm sure there is a connection between the arrhythmias and hiccups."

(26)"I'm 100% convinced that my A-fibs are due to anxiety and lying on my left side."

The varied symptoms are really quite astounding. Once again I can somewhat sympathize with the doctor who hears these many different stories from his atrial fibrillation patients.

On reflection, if I'd discovered the information I've written about in this book on the Internet two years before, I could have saved myself tons of research time, though I don't entirely regret trudging through the deep and sometimes contradictory trenches of medical information.

XI

NO BEDSIDE MANNER

Patient confusion still abounds!!!....and it makes me wonder why the American Heart Association or some other group hasn't done a more extensive statistical analysis of the millions of patients on what actually triggers atrial flutter/fibrillation. There may be a variety of reasons, but what are they?

Even in my small sample (250 people with 212 responses) I've received volumes of extra information that's helped me have a much clearer understanding of this pesky problem and for that matter the whole medical profession.

For example, the comments about how the survey participants were being handled by doctors was very enlightening.

The information in the questionnaires that were returned has left me believing the vast majority of A-fib sufferers feel they're not getting the best treatment or information available, and have resorted to desperately searching the Internet for whatever answers they can come up with.

I firmly believe this is largely due to the confusion and frustration of the doctors themselves. I suspect their frustration manifests itself in many ways since A-fib is often viewed as a nuisance. It follows that if the malady is a nuisance to them, then, I suspect, the patient may be, or soon will be.

These feelings were further highlighted by two recent articles in the *New York Times*. One of them, Abigail Zuger's essay titled, "When the Doctor and Patient Needs Couple's Therapy," reported that Dr. Stephen R. Hahn at the Albert Einstein College of Medicine found in a 1996 survey "that doctors were unenthusiastic about providing care for almost one of every six patients, finding them frustrating and time consuming and not looking forward to their return visits. Not surprisingly, he also found that many of these patients were as unhappy with the care they received as the doctors were unhappy in providing it."

In the same article Dr. William Sledge, a psychiatrist at Yale University School of Medicine in New Haven, said, "Doctors forget that in their interactions with patients both parties show up with baggage from the past that necessarily influences anything they create together."

"After analyzing more than 200 problem-ridden doctor-patient relationships, Dr. Sledge and a colleague, Dr. Alvan Feinstein at Yale, found that simply by advising doctors to ask patients, 'What would you like me to do for you?' at the beginning of every visit, they could vastly improve both parties' satisfaction with the session."

The second story that showed up on the heels of the first, gave me even more to consider when using doctors. This one was vastly more critical of the profession. "It's Enough To Make You Sick, The Way Patients Get Treated," written by Robert Lipsyte, a columnist for the *Times* who is also the author of, "In the Country of Illness: Comfort and Advice for the Journey." Mr. Lipsyte starts his *Times* story by describing a patient, "Sitting naked on tissue paper, mouth dry, heart flip-flopping, clawing at the plastic hide of the examining table. I do not feel as if I'm in a power position. It's been more than 30 minutes and the paper is adhering, shifting with me. My imagination is metastasizing; the syringes, catheters and scalpels in the cabinet all have my name on them. Finally, a fully-dressed human being marches into the room, weary, impatient and, while reading from a folder that really does have my name written on it, demands, 'What seems to be the trouble?'

"If this were a true story, I would mumble, 'I'm really sorry to bother you, doctor, but'.... But since this is a fantasy, I smile confidently as I gesture at a person sitting quietly in a corner and say, 'This is my Patient's Union representative, doctor. You don't mind if we videotape the session.'"

Those who feel they've gone through this sort of treatment will be able to empathize with Mr. Lipsyte's fictional character as well as his next point. He says, "We are frightened and outraged by the tyranny of current health insurance practices. Even when we are lucky enough to have a decent coverage, we often feel trapped in the job that offers it.

"We are frustrated by the decreasing amount of 'face time' with doctors, who themselves admit that the relationship between doctors and patients is critical to getting and staying well. And we are bedeviled by the message of the healer-dealers that somehow we are at fault for being sick; that it is a shame and a punishment, we should be grateful for any mercies the system dispenses."

I have been going to my doctor for some twenty years and I'm pleased to say that there were no problems. During this time, I was also getting my stress test for my heart with him and nothing serious had ever shown up.

Now it's been a little over three years since he discovered I was prone to atrial flutter/fibrillation. It was my first real medical problem, other than the remnants of combat on Pacific islands in World War II. When I think of this doctor I find it difficult to put my finger on why I've never been totally content with his approach. In all probability, if there is any fault in the relationship, the blame most likely lies with me. I've always liked to know precisely what's going on around me, and certainly this applies to my health. After analyzing our relationship, I found that my inability to communicate my concerns to him was an important consideration.

During my business career, I've never been able to put my total confidence in people till I know most of the details of what's behind their thinking, especially if it concerns me or something I'm involved in. For whatever reasons, I think doctors should attempt to figure their patients out and treat each one accordingly as I have with my own clients over the years. This approach has served me quite well.

I've thought as deeply about this aspect of health care as I have about the problem of atrial fib itself. I've attempted to analyze what to do and what I should expect from doctors in the future.

I believe those of us who are older than 50 still expect an entirely different approach to our health care and office procedures than the 50 and under baby boomers. We expect something more like the Dr. Welby type outlined in an earlier chapter.

I, like most people my age, held a deep and abiding respect for the medical profession, the legal profession or any activity that was labeled professional. At one time or another, most older adults have heard of the Hippocratic Oath. To us it denoted dedicated giants who were committed to the integrity of their practice. These pledges set them on pedestals and apart from the general population.

The old movies have their Dr. Kildares, and a array of others who put the patient's care ahead of their own time schedules, money or physical well being. We've all heard the stories of how the old time physicians were paid with chickens or vegetables when money wasn't available.

From this we concluded that a doctor's care of the patient's need was part of his reward for being a doctor. It is with these thoughts that I realize the world we are sliding out of is evolving into a new world we find unreal and difficult to understand.

Over the last few years when one speaks of doctors one invariably mentions the expensive homes they live in, their large expensive cars, and the elaborate parties they give. When the subject does come up about one considering a medical career, it seems invariably the amount of money to be made becomes part of the topic.

From my survey participants' perspective many feel in today's world money has become the paramount consideration for the health care industry, and the patients' care takes a back seat.

This is unlike my old New York City doctor who, upon retiring, *gave* his practice to a young colleague whom he'd carefully selected on the basis of his ability to provide the same care he'd been giving his patients for well over fifty years.

Today, doctoring seems to be a business just like any other with balance sheets and all. They sell them just like others sell insurance agencies or ice cream shops.

Unfortunately, many young persons now coming along seem to be accepting of this. They've been raised during an era that's entirely different from my "older generation".

Therefore, many of us can easily understand why the young doctor who's in the pursuit of wealth is practicing speedy, cubbyhole medicine to make his practice more revenue friendly.

While their incomes are important, the most important aspect of curing any patient is the doctor's knowledge of the whole individual, not just the part that is temporarily broken or diseased.

In retrospect, it's more than foolish to think we can turn back the clock to the way things use to be, and in most cases I'm not sure I'd like to. though with respect to the doctor-patient relationships, and from what I hear, I'm also not so sure public opinion of our medical field will improve till they revisit yesteryear and patients, in general, are treated more like real, live people rather than Blue Cross-Medicare Insurance charges.

As a side issue, I've long believed that a simple remedy to this demeaning problem would be for the insurance companies and Medicare to pay the person who pays for the insurance, then let the insured pay the doctor. I believe this solution isn't possible because of good old American politics. At the very least I feel strongly that physicians and *their staffs* should always remember that patients have paid for the insurance benefits (one way or another) and the carriers paying the doctors and hospitals are only dispensing the patients' money.

XII

YET ANOTHER OPINION

After two years of mixed feelings about the drugs I was taking to eliminate my atrial flutter/fibrillation, I finally made the arduous decision to seek one more opinion. I made several discrete inquiries among friends and acquaintances and learned the name of another highly touted cardiac physician who had a practice in this area. The people I spoke to seemed to believe that Dr. Jon DeSantis was a good bet. He was a few years younger than my present doctor, from the area, and, like my doctor, well-trained and a Fellow in the American College of Cardiology. He had also attended a fine medical school that was highly rated.

My first visit was quite satisfactory. He quickly sized up my need to know. He told me as much as I could expect to hear about the problems of atrial fibrillation. I was glad he made no reference to the other doctor. The other man was an excellent cardiologist, and I'm sure he knew it.

DeSantis believed that atrial fibrillation should be treated aggressively.

He immediately decided that I should see Dr. Brian A. McGovern who was Co-Director of Cardiac Arrhythmia Service at Massachusetts General Hospital/Harvard Medical School, a leading American hospital.

In checking the Internet I discovered his speciality was electrophysiology and he was renowned in the field of atrial fibrillation. It seemed he was just the ticket for me! Everything was moving fast and I liked that. In no time at all I received a call from DeSantis's office establishing a time and date for me to see this specialist.

The following week I made a trip to McGovern's office and spent the better part of two hours with him. The first hour could be described as reviewing history. I gave him all the details from the beginning of the episodes some three years before and from my records I provided him with their frequency and duration. It was more clear to me now after years of researching my problem that this relatively young man knew his subject.

Earlier I'd been told that he was spending one day a week away from his home base at Massachusetts

General Hospital in Boston to visit St. Peters Hospital in Albany, NY, where DeSantis was Chief of Cardiology, instructing other doctors in the art of the ablation technique. My Internet research provided me with additional information. I had learned he was part of a team of doctors who were currently exploring new machinery and techniques to be used during ablation procedures.

The second hour I queried him to find out precisely where I stood. He carefully reviewed with me what I could expect if and when the fibrillation progressed, though at the moment he didn't feel that I had more than lone atrial fibrillation. Most important, he would not recommend a change in my drug therapy until such time as I had documented a normal exercise cardiac perfusion scan. In simple language he explained that this scan would determine if there were any latent or underlying heart disease that the usual stress test would not pick up. If lone atrial fibrillation was verified then he suggested that I go on a drug which is at the upper tolerance level of drugs for the heart.

I had seen the drug mentioned on the Internet and had read that it was suspected of causing many deaths in those people who had underlying heart disease. It became clear to me then why the importance of the exercise perfusion scan.

Naturally my stomach did flip flops knowing the possible consequences of taking the drug, flecainide, or Tambocor®, its trade name.

Nevertheless, I felt that with this doctor I was in good hands and I must have confidence in his abilities if I was to help him lick my problem.

When we parted he mentioned that he would be sending me a complete report. This delighted me for it would help to satisfy my insatiable curiosity about this dilemma.

It was three days later when I received a call from DeSantis's office to set up an appointment in Albany to undergo what the nurse termed "a nuclear stress test." After setting up a date, she briefly explained what this was all about and mentioned that she would send me a confirmation of all the details and what I must do to prepare for it.

The information arrived a couple of days later. It was then I learned that the formal name of the test was "Sestamibi". The letter pointed out that Sestamibi (Cardiolite®) is a chemical attached to a radioactive tracer, technicium. It's given in very small concentrations and is well tolerated by patients. It's a common procedure used to determine how adequate the blood flow is to your heart muscle. The nurse had underscored I should have nothing solid or liquid to eat or drink in the immediate four hours prior to my first visit. Also not to eat food or drink beverages containing caffeine or decaf coffee twelve hours prior to the test. I was instructed to bring comfortable clothing such as a jogging suit and walking shoes. I was told that a nuclear medicine technologist would inject a small amount of this radioactive tracer through a vein in my arm. Then I would be asked to eat a meal to help distribute the Sestamibi properly throughout my system. Upon returning an hour and a half later, thirty minutes of imaging of my heart would be carried out. This would be followed by an echocardiogram. In the afternoon I would be exercised on a tread mill until my heart rate reached an adequate level or I developed symptoms that either I or the staff felt it was necessary to terminate the examination.

While still on the tread mill more nuclear medicine would be injected into my vein and one more minute of exercise would follow. After several delayed minutes for the nuclear medicine to reach maximum levels through the heart, I would then be brought into the nuclear laboratory for another set of images. This whole procedure including lunch would require approximately six hours. The notice stressed that I was not to take my present medicine (Betapace®) the day before or the day of the test.

Without reiterating the actual details of my test, I hasten to add that I began "fibbing" while the echocardiogram was being performed and continued to fib throughout the test and stopped just shortly before leaving the office. In a strange way I was glad the fib had developed, for if there were anything more to my problem they could surely detect it now.

The following Thursday I visited Dr. DeSantis

and he confirmed I had no underlying heart disease. He started me with the recommended regimen of 100mg of Toprol® (metoprolol) and 200mg of Tambocor® (flecainide) a day. In his letter to me Dr. McGovern hadn't explained why he chose this combination of drugs for me, but I was still confident he knew exactly what he was doing.

I made an appointment thirty days later for an assessment as to how these two drugs were working out.

At the moment my psyche had improved immeasurably. While my other doctor was correct in his original assessment of no underlying disease, I was delighted McGovern's more scientific approach took a lot of the educated guess work out of my diagnosis.

Another tremendous improvement in my psyche was a direct result of the excellent treatment afforded me by the cardiologist's staff. It appeared clear to me that the nurse practitioners and general staff had been well schooled in the optimum treatment of a stressed patient. Aside from normal courtesies, they clearly explained every procedure I was involved in and acknowledged the need for patients to understand their treatments.

XIII

THE CURATIVE
MAZE PROCEDURE

Since beginning my investigation of atrial fibrillation and its various treatments, new discoveries seem to be developing much more rapidly than in the past: implantable devices, new more reliable pacemakers, defibrillators, etc. Prominent medical journals are referring to these new procedures almost monthly. After reading an Associated Press wire release written in early 1998 by Lauren Neergaard titled, "Slicing the Heart to Make it Beat," I'm much more receptive to the maze procedure and am looking into it in greater detail, though I must say the accounting given by Neergaard was once again enough to frighten my mule.

The story detailed an invasive technique on a 56 year old patient from Albany, Georgia, developed by Dr.

James L. Cox, of Georgetown University Hospital, Professor and Chairman, Cardiovascular and Thoracic Surgery, Surgical Director, Georgetown Cardiovascular Institute, and the nationally recognized guru as the originator of the open heart maze procedure. This invasive technique is being discussed in some circles as the only permanent cure for atrial fibrillation. The technique has undergone major modifications since 1987 and is now referred to as the Maze III procedure. It has been in continuous use since 1992.

Using the open heart method, Dr. Cox has operated on 346 patients in the last ten years with a high degree of success. Of these, there has been only a four percent relapse and those cases were mild enough for drug therapy.

Now it appears that in some patients surgeons don't need to cut open your chest and breastbone to get to the heart to perform the maze procedure. Advances in technology and surgical instrumentation make it possible to do the procedure through smaller incisions in the chest wall depending on the individual's body shape and size. Apparently large chested persons (such as myself) may be ruled.

Until the time of Neergaard's article, Dr. Cox had done only twelve patients with this less invasive procedure and couldn't yet predict long term results. However, several of these patients were up and pain free in days.

One, another cardiac surgeon, was strong enough a week later to stand seven hours at Cox's elbow, studying how to do the surgery. Cox jokes, "You know with minimal invasive surgery you send the patient to recovery and the doctor to intensive care."

My previous reluctance to consider this as an option was that I didn't believe I was mentally prepared for full blown open heart surgery as Cox's original maze procedure called for.

Obviously I was most curious why all the cuts to the heart. In pursuing the answer during my follow-up investigation, I learned that Dr. Cox was formerly associated with Washington School of Medicine, Barnes Hospital in St. Louis, Missouri. It was there that he began this development, placing electrodes on beating hearts and discovered in atrial fibrillation, electrical impulses become chaotic. They twirl in circles like small tornadoes instead of following an ordinary route from the atria, the heart's top chambers, down into the main pumping chambers, the ventricles. Apparently his task was to prevent the electrical currents from tail-spinning. If he could prevent the tail spins, atrial fibrillation could be eliminated. He faced the $64 question on how. "Scar tissue will never conduct electrical activity. It is the perfect insulator," Cox explained.

Subsequently, Cox devised cuts (scar tissue) on the heart that would guide electrical current along one path into the atria, then give it a way out, plus a few blind alleys, small detours to activate all sides of the heart muscle.

Neergaard went on to say that Dr. Cox isn't alone in trying a less invasive technique; doctors who learn the procedure from him are experimenting, too. "What Jimmy Cox has done has been truly revolutionary," said Dr. Andrew Epstein of the University of Alabama, Birmingham. "We're hoping to find better ways of doing it with a catheter."

In earlier experiments with radiofrequency ablation, doctors were threading lasers through catheters to burn the pattern into the heart instead of cutting it. Cox is highly skeptical; he'd repaired the hearts of some patients with deep cardiac tissue burns. For now Epstein cautions potential patients to seek specialists. "It is just not the kind of procedure that is going to be done in everybody's backyard."

Subsequent to Lauren Neergaard's article, I contacted Ms. Terry Palazzo, Dr. Cox's Nurse Specialist, Cardiovascular and Thoracic Surgery. She was kind enough to forward to me a complete package of material that helped satisfy most of my questions. Later she was most gracious in providing me with the names of patients who had had the maze procedure performed. I spoke by phone to four of them (three had had the open heart procedure and one the newer less invasive procedure). All of them had nothing but high praise for Dr. Cox and his staff.

THE CURATIVE MAZE PROCEDURE

To avoid belaboring the point, in summary, I asked each patient how they felt about the procedure and was their operation successful? All said yes. In spite of some minor problems that each had been warned about in advance, they were now doing extremely well and felt it was the only way to go. Each of them had exhausted the drug regimen. In one case the participant had been through seven anti-arrhythmic drugs to no avail. Interestingly, the seven drugs were insisted on by his insurance company before they would pay for the maze operation.

As I pursued the maze technique, I found myself with some very serious questions about why in the world I'm even bothering taking drugs and whether in the long run the side effects are destroying my liver, kidneys and heart with no lasting benefit. It appears to me that some of us on drug regimens should, if they qualify, immediately consider the radiofrequency ablation or the maze procedure.

After much research and in my view, Dr. James L. Cox is truly a man to be admired and if there is anybody he could be compared with I would think it could be Dr. Michael D. DeBakey, who at the age of 90 is one of America's legendary, all time great vascular surgeons. It seems that Dr. Cox has advanced the art of electrophysiology and the maze technique as thoroughly as Dr. DeBakey has advanced the technology of vascular grafts, and improved the recovery from arterial bypass surgery.

As recently as May of 2000, I was in touch with Dr. Cox's office and they were again kind enough to bring me up to date on all the details of his maze procedure's outcome. Since September of 1987, Dr. Cox has performed the Maze procedure on 346 patients, 65 of whom had the minimally invasive procedure. He has seen a 100 percent cure of atrial fibrillation in these patients (97 percent without drug therapy and only 3 percent with drugs).

Dr. Cox's Nurse Specialist, Terry Palazzo, has created a Web site:

(http://members.aol.com/mazern/index.htm)

and offers a packet that can be printed from the Web site titled, "What You Need To Know about AF and The Maze Procedure."

In addition to Cox's successes, Dr. Patrick McCarthy of the Cleveland Clinic Foundation has also performed the Maze procedure on 100 patients, from 1991 to June of 1999. A recent paper written by him in "Seminars in Thoracic and Cardiovascular Surgery ", Vol. 12, No.1 (January 2000, pp 25-29) provides his statistics.

U.S. New and World Report, in their annual guide to America's Best Hospitals, ranks The Cleveland Clinic as number one in cardiology and cardiac surgery. The very fact that they are performing this procedure indicates to me that it is no longer experimental and is definitely here to stay.

Rather than paraphrase a recent patient's survey letter to me concerning Dr. Cox and the maze, I'm entering it here so readers can draw their own conclusions.

"I am a 38 year old female with a 15 year history of atrial fibrillation/flutter.

"My descent into arrhythmia began as a small series of "flutter-like" movements in my chest. I was concerned, but I was also 23 years old and at that age you feel that only kryptonite can bring you down. I didn't seek treatment for four years.

"It was due to a hospitalization for a totally unrelated cause that they were finally able to catch my a fib on an EKG.

"So started the long, long road of medications that didn't work, a heart condition that progressed over the years to the point where I was having daily attacks, gaining weight and literally losing any lust for life.

"In 1990 I was hospitalized with an irregular heartbeat of 220. For the three previous years, I had been medicated with Lanoxin and a short try with Verapamil and Inderal. They all failed to control the arrhythmia and the rate.

"My doctors started experimenting on me with fervor. I ran the gamut from Norpace to Ethmozine to Rythmol and more. Nothing would stop the "flopping fish" effect of my heart and nothing brought me any relief.

"The closest I got to being able to function was a combination of Sectral (a beta-blocker) and Lanoxin (Digoxin). I was on those for years. They didn't stop the attacks, but they kept the rate below 120 and kept me out of the emergency room.

"The episodes got more and more debilitating over the years. I started having them three to four times a week. And I got more lethargic and more depressed.

"Enter the Maze. By the time I heard about the Maze, I had given up hope that anything was going to help me. I was on the last chance drug, Amiodarone, and it was doing nothing but making it worse.

"I was watching my children grow up from my prone position on the couch. My husband had become not only the breadwinner, but the housekeeper, too. I felt useless, tired and my despair deepened each day.

"To say that the Maze was a shining beacon at the end of a dark tunnel is not overstating the matter. I found the surgery on a message board (the Internet) for arrhythmias. I called Dr. Cox's office in Georgetown and got all the information available. In two days I had made my decision, sent the office my medical records, started the six-week battle with my insurance company and was finally allowing myself a bit of optimism that maybe there WAS something out there that would finally allow me to live a normal life again.

"I had the surgery May 5th, 1999. Dr. Cox not

only saved my life (deep down I always carried the knowledge that I wouldn't live to ripe old age, but this surgery changed that, too), but he gave me my life back! I know that this all came about because God led me, stepping stone by stepping stone, to Dr. Cox. I had prayed that a miracle would come along to make me "normal" and God answered me with Dr. Cox.

"And what an answer! I've been afib/flutter free since my surgery and I feel wonderful!! It wasn't an easy thing to go through. The psychological effects are traumatic and the physical effects are debilitating. But I now have a future filled with hope. I can dream my dreams and know that with God's help I can make them come true. It doesn't get any better than this."
Signed: Lisa

In a later interview on the telephone, she informed me that she would be happy to discuss her experience with anyone interested in the Maze.

I will be covering other new developments in cardiac rhythm management as they relate to atrial fibrillation/flutter in a later chapter.

XIV

FOOD FOR THOUGHT

I guess if anybody has tried to find a workable formula to stop atrial fib, I have. While researching drugs, radiofrequency ablation and the maze procedure, I've also paid close attention to all of the articles I've come across about foods and vitamins that might help the heart and put an end to this ever present nuisance. Unfortunately, I haven't found anything that was a magic bullet, though I believe the life style changes I've made have indeed paid out in the long run.

In my more positive moments I recall with some glee that it wasn't too many years ago (about 25) that most doctors pooh-poohed vitamin supplements. When asked about them they generally answered, "I'm not sure they'll help you, but if you feel better taking them, go ahead." At that time I believe there was more respect for their opinions and I venture to guess that most of their patients chose to accept their doctors' words as more negative than not. As a result, they avoided the cost and inconvenience of vitamin supplements but may also have missed out on some important health benefits.

Years ago I began paying much closer attention to vitamins after one of my employees had a heart attack at 45 and not too long afterwards was up and around and doing great without the availability of bypass surgery. He seemed to believe that his improved health was mainly due to a new discovery he had read about a few years earlier in *Prevention Magazine*.

While we were visiting in my office in New York one day, he began to extol the virtues of Vitamin E and Vitamin C that he found in the form of rose hips, that little red ball that almost anyone can see in the fall of the year on a particular type of rose bush. There were lots of them at our lodge in the Adirondacks. His health and condition seemed to improve so rapidly that I began to think there was something to it and it wasn't long after that I began to consume 400 mg of E and 500 mg of C a day. While I hadn't had a heart attack, he had touted the E as super good for circulation. To his credit he retired at 75 and at 86 is still alive and kicking with his original heart.

Over the years I have watched the acceptance of vitamins grow to such an extent that I, like thousands of other individuals, have been taking recommended doses of many, such as a multiple vitamin stress tablet.

While I suspect they have really helped me, my general attitude is that for the few dollars I spend per week for these entities, I strongly believe they're clearly worth the money.

Along the way I've witnessed some pretty wild claims to what various vitamin supplements and home remedies can do for one. For example Laetrile comes to mind. Laetrile, as defined by Webster's dictionary, is the name of a chemical made primarily from an extract of apricot pits, used by some in the belief that it is an anti-neoplastic agent.

The chemical made national news about 20 years ago. I remember it so vividly because a child who was suffering from cancer lived only 20 miles or so from our summer home in upstate New York. The mother was valiantly fighting the medical profession, the State Health Department, and anyone else who challenged her right to avail her child of this treatment. Overnight a cottage industry sprang up in Mexico and great streams of Americans paraded in and out of that country's clinics in the hope that this was a miracle cure.

Steve McQueen, one of my all time favorite movie actors, was one of those Americans and needless to say he attracted hundreds of newsmen who reported the story internationally.

I remember clearly recalling that it was only the people who had the problem who were willing to spend almost anything to cure cancer or for that matter any life threatening disease that afflicts them.

When I asked the American Cancer Society about Laetrile, their official view was, "After study of literature and available information, ACS has found no evidence that Laetrile results in objective benefits in the treatment of cancer in human beings." Both McQueen and the child subsequently died.

Those of us at the time who didn't suffer the problem followed the stories with skepticism and felt just a little sorry for the people who were sucked into the traps of greedy charlatans. Those and many cure-alls like them, with the help of the media, often turned alternative cures into shams and pushed a lot of us away from anything but good old meat and potatoes and cereal and ice cream.

Now things are different. Twenty-five years has jumped us into discoveries that we thought we'd never see. Along with astronomical advances in bypass surgery, the knowledge of cholesterol and its damage to the arteries, miracle drugs that have cured everything from polio to measles have astounded us. Along with this, quantum leaps have occurred in the minds of doctors and their willingness to accept the fact that drug companies are not the only ones who have important answers, though many of us still believe that if it isn't sanctioned by the Food and Drug Administration it is probably bad for us.

The mid-90s brought hundreds of new wellness

centers, homeopathic doctors and the likes (they are springing up like McDonalds and Wal-Marts), most of which are taking up the slack that's generated by a national uneasiness about HMOs and conventional health care.

To compound this, a headlined Associated Press story out of Washington, D. C. reported on a story in the *Journal of the American Medical Association*. "AMA says some Chinese herbal remedies are okay." When one reads further they report that "an estimated four out of every ten Americans now try, the *Journal* judged, alternative remedies that were subjected to strict scientific study - and found that just like in conventional medicine, some work and some don't."

They found that Chinese herbs helped irritable bowel disease that Western medicine doesn't always relieve and that saw palmetto seems to shrink enlarged prostates.

Then they add the bizarre finding that heating the herb mugwort next to the little toe of a pregnant woman to help turn her baby out of the risky breach position really works and the *Journal* recommends that Western women try it.

I no longer feel so much out of step when I'm searching the Internet for alternative medicine to supplement my current knowledge of what is available through regular channels.

In a recent article in the *Washington Post* titled,

"Educated Seek Alternate Cures", the writer pointed out that "People who seek care from alternative medicine tend to be better educated than medical main streamers according to a national survey. Forty percent of respondents said they had used some form of alternative health care during the previous year." Use of alternative health care was defined by the survey as use in the past year of treatments such as acupuncture, homeopathy, herbal therapy, chiropractic massage, and high dose mega vitamins.

The survey was based on a detailed questionnaire sent at random to 1500 Americans. It was initiated by John A. Astin, a researcher at Stanford University School of Medicine in Palo Alto, California. His results were reported in the *Journal of the American Medical Association.* Users of this type treatment had equal percentages of people who were highly satisfied or highly dissatisfied with mainstream medicine. Such factors as age, gender, race, ethnicity made no difference in the survey.

Since I am one of the many Americans who have been looking at how food and alternative medicines have been increasingly accepted, I was further interested by Jane Brody's column in the *New York Times,* "Alternative Medicine Makes Inroads, But Watch Out For Curves," that seems to confirm Mr. Astin's points. She clearly says, and uses charts to boot, that 42 percent of American adults use some kind of alternative care and states that it is the largest growth industry in health care today. Of some 1500 adults, 44 percent said they would use an alternative method if traditional medical care was not producing the desired results. "While most doctors shun such care and question its merits and reliability, Americans are voting with their feet and pocketbooks. Studies have shown that patients make more visits each year to alternative care practitioners than to primary care physicians and most of them pay out of their own pockets for the care they receive."

Several months ago Nancy Beth Jackson, of the *New York Times*, wrote an article, " Doctors' Warning: Beware of Herbs Side Effects," that particularly attracted my attention. It concerned a 58 year old North Carolina heart patient who had combined, with the use of his prescription drug, the herbal remedy, valerin. It is a root that sometimes is called "nature's tranquilizer." "His self administered treatment led to unexpected cardiac complications and delirium after a surgical biopsy of a lung nodule. The problem was not that he had taken valerin, but that he had stopped. Unexpected withdrawal symptoms put him in intensive care. The patient survived - and no longer takes valerin for sleeplessness. Like prescription drugs, herbal products act like chemicals in the body and may cause the same kinds of side effects, withdrawal symptoms, and interactions, warned the doctors who linked the heart crisis to valerin.

"A lot of people don't think of herbs as medicines," said Dr. P. Murali Doraiswamy, of the Duke University Medical Center.

An article in the *Archives of Family Medicine* states that one-third of Americans use one herb or another, but often haven't any information about their safety.

While I'm not prone to challenging the medical profession by searching for some witch doctor who guarantees he can cure everything from heart disease to cancer, I decided to closely examine recommendations from all creditable sources about foods, vitamins or herbs that will improve my general health.

For example, a few months ago I read that the *Harvard Heart Letter* was recommending eating more of certain types of fish. Those fish in particular contain more omega-3 fatty acids. Shortly after reading this I came across the *Medical Tribune* (Family Physician edition) on the Internet reporting that "according to researchers from Harvard Medical School and Brigham and Women's Hospital, both of Boston, men who reported eating fish (mackerel, blue fish, salmon, tuna, white fish, shrimp and lobster) at least once a week had had half the risk of sudden cardiac death compared with men who reported eating fish less than once a month." The physicians' health study had questioned an impressive 20,550 men to determine these results.

A similar story was released by Mayo Clinic and during the past few months dozens of others. Since it has long been known that the Japanese consume millions of tons of these kinds of fish annually and it is well known that they have the lowest risk of heart disease of any nation in the world, I stand more than convinced and have included fish in my diet once or twice a week.

Another benefit of eating fish is that it has helped me maintain my weight at a consistent level after losing 48 pounds during the past two years.

In many ways I've enjoyed researching this material. I'm sure most of us know the old adage "an apple a day keeps the doctor away" and by extension if you can keep the doctor away you can prolong your life. Also you're less likely to be subject to the risk of medical mistakes. I mention this because the other findings that result in better health tout fruits and vegetables and though I've never been prone to eating many vegetables, I've stepped up my consumption of fruit at least twenty-fold. I'm fast developing an attitude that I'd rather have a fresh glass of orange juice, a beautifully ripened peach or some nice California grapes, than I would so many of the other sweets that I've enjoyed in the past. I have substituted no-fat frozen yogurt for ice cream and I find I now like it almost as well, though my wife and I occasionally go out during an afternoon and indulge ourselves in cones of high fat ice cream. We've learned over time that the best of foods can be boring if eaten too frequently and we try to pace ourselves accordingly.

Once again, in Jane Brody's Personal Health column in the *New York Times*, in the article, "Pass the Wine and Olive Oil and Other Lessons from Crete," she tells a story of 12,000 men in 7 countries studied in 1960 by Dr. Ancel Keys, where he found those least likely to develop heart disease lived on the Isle of Crete. His co-investigator, Dr. Henry Blackburn, Professor Emeritus at the University of Minnesota, has written that the low-risk Cretan is a sheep herder or small farmer, a bee keeper or fisherman, or a tender of olives or vines, who walks to work daily. His mid-day main meal is of eggplant with large mushrooms, crisp vegetables, country bread dipped in olive oil. Included in this weekly diet is an occasional bit of lamb, then a bit of chicken, and twice a week there is fresh fish from the sea. They always consume a sharp local wine that completes the meal.

Most of us can figure out why this might be the ideal diet, and we should be able to follow it because of America's wonderful array of supermarket foods.

In contrast we, as well as our kids and grandkids, are bombarded daily with beautiful television ads of Big Macs and fries. Television inundates adults with cooking shows from the world over, and we are further tempted with an infinite variety of new dishes offered in restaurants.

With respect to vitamin supplements I suspect they are responsible for my improved energy levels and thereby are helping my heart, though I'm quick to add the manufacturers are blessed with the fact that if you stay well you're apt to lay it to the vitamins and if you fall ill it "couldn't be the vitamins," unless of course you're into mega doses.

At this point in my life I've tried to be as careful as humanly possible in those I consume. I've also tried not to go wild consuming one of everything in the health food stores. Consequently I'm down to a daily dose of a multi-vitamin stress tab, vitamins C, E, B 6 and 12, magnesium, and folic acid. I also take CoQ10 which a lot of people may not have heard of. I know I hadn't until a few months ago while surfing the Internet. A person who professes to be suffering from A fib and swears it has made a difference, recommended it and then sent me some literature. Apparently it is an enzyme that purports to strengthen the normal heart muscle and is consumed in great quantities in Japan where it was developed. Again, knowing that the rate of heart disease there is the lowest in the world, I decided that the additional cost would not deter me.

My final conclusions are that if each one of these vitamins have been sufficiently recognized by creditable sources and that I suffer no obvious side effects from them, then they are worth a shot. With respect to the vitamins I'm taking I've seen them all touted highly in various creditable publications.

However, to add further confusion to a raft of

already complex information, the Consumers League, with the help of the Food and Drug Administration, has recently published a brochure listing drug-food combinations patients should avoid such as grapefruit and calcium-channel blockers, high doses of vitamin E with Coumadin®, and coffee or colas with Tagamet®, Zantac® and Pepcid®

By way of extension, one must consider that everything we eat is in effect a chemical compound. Which ones are truly best for each individual, is anyone's guess. I've let my body be my guide.

XV

IS IT A SHELL GAME?

I often think about how long it's been since I first experienced atrial fibrillation.

Two months after its discovery I was truly amazed I was still alive and kicking and without the horrific results of a stroke.

In the very beginning I repeatedly ran across the following medical caveat concerning the malady. "<u>The incidence of stroke is much greater in people with A-fib than the general population.</u>" I've continued to be dismayed to see medical bulletins point out that stroke and heart attacks were the leading health killers in the U.S. if their statistics can be believed. (In other words, A-fibs are not life threatening, just stroke threatening.) I had never remotely considered I'd be a candidate for either.

I was troubled deciding which I'd rather have, death or a disabling stroke, as if I had a choice. With death that's the end of my problem. With a stroke, it's just the beginning of a huge burden for my wife. Unfortunately this hideous disability could last for many years. The thought of dragging around a leg or a worthless arm with slurred, or no speech at all is definitely the pits. That's what happened to my brother which naturally increases my anxiety.

After much research I happily concluded that lone A-fib didn't quite fit in the highest risk category of those with other underlying heart problems though there is still an additional risk. It was then I decided to summarize all that I'd learned during the past three years, assess what my doctors had prescribed that had helped me and what I'd discovered on my own and applied to myself that may have helped. And I've helped myself a lot, though at the moment I do credit both sides about fifty-fifty.

Many years before as a management consultant I'd practiced a technique of cross-checking the words of corporate managers. I'd learned its value. This exercise was applied mostly to chief executive officers and their vice presidents. It seemed the brighter the executives, the more difficult it was to find out what was truly on their minds. With most ambitious executives, they wanted their cake and to eat it, too.

From this perspective I've learned most physicians are intellectually brighter than corporate managers. Though I know now they know less about human nature than a good corporate sales executive.

I had trouble coming to grips with the thought that a great majority of them haven't the foggiest idea of the actual cause of lone atrial fibrillation or which drug will put it in check. I very much wanted to believe they were all-knowing on all medical subjects.

With A-fib I'm certain it's still a hit or miss game and patients like me are a bit like guinea pigs. For this ailment there are about twenty marketed drugs and not all of them are approved for my particular condition. I was changed from one to another every few months without any true benefit, and I'm certain in some cases the drugs even made my condition worse.

I truly believe doctors served me best by unintentionally pointing me in directions that I could explore on my own. I am having fewer episodes with shorter durations by applying techniques I've gleaned from a litany of medical publications.

The American Heart Association in a current clinical trial is just now trying to determine if the drugs they prescribe for atrial fibrillation really serve a benefit to the patients, the same as the AFFIRM study. In retrospect it would have helped me immensely if I'd been warned that this uncertainty was the case from the very beginning, but I wasn't.

With respect to the doctors I've met, I truly feel they think they do the best they can to care for the patients' needs, though I have no doubt the current practices of the HMO's, Medicare, Medicaid, private and public health insurance companies give them a fit with frustrating regimentation when dictating what they can or cannot charge. Unfortunately the patient is squarely in the middle of the fracas and this shouldn't be. It's bound to have a negative impact on doctor-patient relationships.

As most people know, attempting to be one's own lawyer is to be represented by a fool. Likewise, being one's own doctor is equally as foolish, though I've now confirmed there are many things that can be done to assist the doctor in his quest to help the patient.

First, I had to face up to the fact that doctors don't have as much time as I'd like for them to think about my particular problem. I also suspect, from the way they rush around from examining room to examining room, they don't have time to pre-review my chart or think about me till I'm in one of their little cubby holes striped to the waist, weighed, with blood pressure taken by an assistant. There I sit patiently waiting for the doctor to show up.

In this modern, fast moving and highly charged age of distrusted medicine, doctors must answer to many different groups concerning the patient's care. In my case, they answer to Medicare as well as Blue Cross and not to me even though I paid for the insurance. In others it's an HMO or another private insurance company.

If they help the indigent, treatment is paid for by

a bureaucratic run state Medicaid agency. They also live under constant threats of frivolous and real malpractice suits.

These organizations are all competing for their time and attention. Worst yet, more often than not, these third party payers want to control their practices and income by regulating how much time can be spent with a patient, what treatment can be given and how much they will pay the doctor for these services. The corporations and governments are motivated to reduce fees so more profits or savings can remain in *their own pockets and in many cases with little or no concern for the patient.*

Under these pressured and intense circumstances, doctors, like all the rest of us, are prone to mistakes, as pointed out in a recent report from the National Academy of Science though here my concern is that they're dispensing drugs that can have significant side effects which can be and often are life threatening. The wrong drug can be as deadly as an eighteen wheel truck running a red light and broadsiding an innocent passenger car. The thought of surviving a crash like this doesn't leave much to the imagination. However, the truck is clearly at fault and the police, with witnesses, can easily verify it. If the doctor makes a mistake prescribing the wrong or too much drug, and one dies, who's to know.

Mistakes are bound to happen. After all, in 1997,

according to IMS Health, Inc., the public spent the humongous sum of $79.8 billion for prescription drugs and that was up from $37.7 billion in 1990. There are 56,000 full time sales representatives from the top 40 pharmaceutical companies calling on doctors to make their sales pitches and annual quotas, so said the Scott-Levin consulting firm of Pennsylvania. Scott-Levin estimates that pharmaceutical companies in the United States spent $5.3 billion dollars in the first 11 months of 1998 sending representatives into doctors' offices and hospitals. This equates to nearly 1 salesperson and near-ly $100,000 for every group of 11 practicing physicians in the country, a size and budget that any educational venture would be jealous of.

Moreover, the *Journal of the American Medical Association* found in one of its studies published in 1995 that in tape recordings of thirteen presentations by pharmaceutical salesmen, a dozen errors of fact were made by these representatives to doctors, errors that invariably favored the presenter's own drug over the competition.

It seems to me that many of these company rep-resentatives care not what they say to get the doctor to keep on writing prescriptions for their drugs. I personal-ly have known of several drug firms that have rewarded doctors with expensive gifts (VCRs and cameras for instance) for writing a certain number of prescriptions of their drug. And I presume that the salesman is equally rewarded if he produces an increase in his doctors' prescriptions.

As I mentioned earlier, there's little wonder that over 100,000 patients die of the wrong drug or a drug overdose each year. That's twice as many as are killed in automobile accidents annually. For a better perspective on these numbers, there were approximately 400,000 Americans killed in World War II over a three and half year period.

Recently the *New England Journal of Medicine* published a paper by three prominent doctors, Dr. Raymond Woosley of Georgetown University, Dr. J. J. Wood and Dr. C. Michael Stein, both of Vanderbilt University in Nashville. They suggested that the United States needed an independent drug safety agency analogous to the transportation board to investigate drugs that "crashed" as well as a mandatory reporting system that would catch adverse drug reaction as early as possible.

It's hard to believe that such an agency does not already exist. The FDA is supposed to do this but I assume Congressional politics doesn't allow them enough money to fund this very important public need.

While my two following examples are not about bad drugs themselves, I believe it's equally as important there be another agency for patients or their families to report unfavorable incidents.

Currently when a drug harms an individual patient, and since there is no specific public agency to investigate this, I firmly believe leaving the reporting to the doctor is like having the fox guard the proverbial hen house.

If, for no other reason, an independent agency would help keep the doctors on their toes as well as keeping more unsuspecting patients alive.

One highly respected cardiologist abruptly took me off a beta-blocker. All that I've researched tells me that one should be taken off this drug on a *gradual basis*. I assumed he knew what he was doing and didn't question this change to another drug.

Later when my episodes increased and I began taking Coumadin®, I had to take a weekly blood test till the right level in my blood was achieved. Then, when I reached it, I had to continue with a monthly test till I no longer needed the drug. I was informed by my friend, Dr. John Mullane, who worked on Coumadin® for DuPont Pharmaceuticals, that the desired level of Coumadin® in the blood was between 2.0 and 3.0. If its INR (International Normalized Ratio) is higher, 4.0 or above, it is associated with a higher risk of bleeding. It can even be life threatening. Much more serious internal bleeding can result from bad falls that many older people seem to be plagued with.

While traveling in the South, I was surprised when my INR range changed from too much Vitamin K in my diet. I was eating too many beans, collards and other green leafy vegetables.

However, it wasn't long before I discovered the real danger in this blood thinner. It seemed to me to be more in the drawing of the blood to be tested than in the effects of the drug levels in my body.

DeSantis's nurse and the Glens Falls hospital handled this important step properly. The hospital was careful with the paper work. The labels for the blood work were computer generated. The lab was clean and bright. The technician was pleasant and very efficient, all of which one expects.

While traveling away from home I searched for a duplicate of my local hospital blood lab. With only one exception, (The Mayo Clinic in Jacksonville, Florida) I had some very hairy experiences with what I would deem to be careless technicians. In some cases they jabbed me in a muscle several times before finding my vein. My arm was unusually sore for several days. In one lab they failed to swab my arm with alcohol before inserting the needle. Cleaning germs from the area where the needle enters the vein, I'm told, is quite important.

In another, I had to have the test redone because the lab that analyzes the sample found clots in the tube.

Two more were very disorganized and confused and I feared they'd label my blood improperly. I later learned that in most states these technicians are required to be recertified every year. In most cases the laboratories appeared to me to be disasters waiting to happen for some unsuspecting soul. In the end I chalked up their performances to boredom and lack of proper supervision. And my research indicates there are many other obscure technical inaccuracies floating around in the medical industry.

Despite all the scares I've had with the drawing of blood, my own feelings are that anyone who has had atrial flutter/fibrillation or any malady that may suggest a stroke, should remain on Coumadin® for life, which I plan to do.

XVI

THE FACTS OF DEATH

R ecently, Dr. Lawrence Altman wrote in the *New York Times,* Science section, a column titled, "Getting it Right on the Facts of Death." The information he revealed was most disturbing. He reported, "The autopsy rate has plummeted to less than 10% from about 50% in the 1960's. Apparently, *coronary artery disease* is the default diagnosis for the death certificate when doctors are not sure of the cause of death. Despite the importance of the death certificate, the message about the frequent flaws is unpopular in medical circles because it implicitly criticizes medical education and practice. Studies in the United States and elsewhere have documented varying degrees of inaccuracy in death certificate information with some showing an error rate of 30% to 40%."

As I read his column I shuddered to think of all

those poor souls who died without anyone really knowing the real reason for their demise, not to mention the impact on future generations when they attempt for the benefit of genetics to identify the causes of their parents' deaths.

I can understand this frustration since my father died when I was only three and according to undocumented, passed-down information, he could have died of anything from gangrene as the result of an accident to a heart attack. The death certificate is questionable. In any case I have no real idea. And similar circumstances took place when, a little later, my mother passed on. There is no concrete evidence that it was her heart which killed her. It would be very beneficial to me and my four children, as well as to my doctors, if we knew the facts of their deaths as opposed to flimsy rumors. I've often heard, and I vaguely remember, when my mother was young she complained about having a heart condition. Was she in fact plagued with atrial fibrillation? Since starting this book I've asked myself many times, where in the medical profession (as there are in all other professions) are all the checks and balances, or don't they apply to this hallowed group? All hospitals have committees which review deaths and serious complications. Presumably, there is some variability in their diligence, but often there is no oversight of actions that occur in an office practice which doesn't result in a hospital admission.

When autopsies are performed changes in death certificates are allowed, though frequently the information is not forwarded or the certificate changed.

Dr. Altman continued, "Doctors have been required to sign death certificates in all states since at least 1933. Yet formal instruction on how to assign a cause of death is spotty. Instead, the learning generally comes informally during residency training when doctors may ask colleagues, 'How do I fill this thing out?'" He goes on to say that this question is often answered by other doctors, or nurses, or medical records workers or even occasionally funeral directors. And who's to say how much funeral directors knew about the health of the deceased.

For all we know heart disease may be less deadly than cancer, since many statistics on this disease are based on inaccurate information on death certificates. It's just a more convenient entry for the doctors that isn't likely to be challenged.

It all sounds like material for a good "who done it," murder mystery.

XVII

GOD HELPS
THOSE WHO HELP
THEMSELVES

For many of the reasons I've discovered during my quest to become all informed about my heart, as you can see in the past chapters, I've concentrated on helping myself live a bit longer and stop depending entirely on my doctors, though I still intend to see them regularly and continue with my drugs.

As a result of my conclusions, I honestly believe, as I've said earlier, I have vastly improved my health by eating well, eliminating stress and developing a more positive attitude about the progress that is being made in the heart disease field. I feel more comfortable knowing that under certain circumstances there is indeed life after atrial fibrillation.

My front line troops are made up of the following bodyguards:

Stress:

I'm now positively convinced that stress can indeed play a major role in the management of atrial fibrillation. In the beginning I was more than convinced that I was devoid of anything relating to this. I thought I had the world by the tail till this elusive and misbehaving heart problem showed up.

After much time and analysis I began to realize that A-fib itself was creating a very high level of stress. Just waiting on pins and needles for another episode to begin would set my pulse racing. It wasn't until I began to tell myself that the episodes were going to continue to be a part of my life and there was so damn little I could do about them that I came to grips with my mortality.

In the beginning it wasn't easy. As I've said, I was constantly reminding myself that while in A-fib I could have a stroke or even die. Finally I acknowledged that for everyone death is inevitable and it's just a matter of time before we all go. There seemed to be comfort knowing I wasn't the only one singled out. Since my affairs were in order and my wife would be well provided for, I began eliminating my stress when I decided there was no point in dying more than once.

Weight adjustment:

As I've said, I've lost nearly fifty pounds during

the last three and a half years, though I'm not entirely sure if my blood pressure has dropped because of the medication or the tremendous loss of weight. Maybe it's both. No matter, I feel better and since the world, including all doctors, thinks it's good, I'm happy I've been able to accomplish it in spite of my continued exposure to good food.

Exercise:

I walk about two and a half to three miles each day. It took a while but now I enjoy these walks, especially when my wife and dog accompany me. I mostly live on the second floor of my house with my den on the first floor. I've finally gotten used to trekking from one floor to the other at least fifteen times a day when I want something such as my glasses. It seems that everything is always on the other floor. I'm consoled by knowing that this extra exercise is definitely good for my health, though a recent study (1/28/99), published in the Journal *of the American Medical Association*, found that "yuppies" gain little more benefit from strenuous exercise when compared to less active people who were not quite couch potatoes.

The Cooper Institute of Aerobics Research in Dallas study followed 235 men and women between the ages 35 and 60 who were divided into two groups and monitored for two years. One group spent 20 to 60 minutes vigorously exercising up to five days a week. The other incorporated 30 minutes a day of "lifestyle" exercise. At the end of six months the "lifestyle" group (normal everyday activity as opposed to complete sedentary immobility) did just as well in the improvement of their cholesterol ratios, blood pressure and body fat. I no longer feel embarrassed when a yuppie passes me in the park running like a young antelope right out of the wilds of Africa.

Eating heart healthy foods:

Many years ago the caretaker at our lodge, said at least once a day, "We are what we eat." Roland was a devoted eater and among his favorite foods was bacon that was hardly cooked. Unfortunately he died at the age of 62, by today's standards a relatively young man, and the cause of death as it was later reported was a massive heart attack brought on by plugged up arteries. Even before I found myself with atrial fib I was quite conscious of his eating habits and had cut back drastically on my breakfast bacon. When I do indulge I enjoy it only if it is thoroughly cooked and drained of most fat. This part of my self-help regimen was not too hard, especially since I already enjoy most of the foods recommended by the major heart institutes (Framingham, Harvard Medical School, Johns Hopkins Hospital, Mayo and Cleveland Clinics).

At least once a week I have fish with high levels of Omega-3 oils recommended by the nutrition experts. Trout, salmon, tuna, shrimp, lobster, and many other ocean going fish have this magic oil. After all, as I said earlier, if the Japanese survive on fish and have the world's lowest heart disease per capita, then there must be something to it.

As an added incentive, the Harvard Heart Letter recently reported that oily fish with this Omega-3, eaten once a week, will <u>specifically help toward eliminating atrial fibrillation</u>. And obviously I'm all for that.

As for the next self-imposed treatment, my dear old grandmother would have exclaimed. "Heavens to Betsy, that sounds like a great idea."

<u>Eating Chocolate</u>:

I was happily amused when I read in the respected British medical journal, *Lancet,* that eating chocolate helped males live longer. *Lancet* went on to say that they couldn't explain this phenomenon. They speculated, however, that antioxidants present in chocolate might have a health benefit. In a study of 7,841 Harvard male graduates they found that chocolate and candy eaters lived almost a year longer than those who abstained, though I can't help but wonder if Nestle or the makers of Dutch chocolate weren't behind the study. Apparently dark chocolate contains approximately four times the amount of catechins as tea, the operative antioxidant we are all looking for.

As an added incentive to me, my mother-in-law, who lived to the ripe old age of 96, sucked on hard candy and ate chocolates almost every day. She was skinny as a rail and lively to the end.

Scientists have long since discovered that chocolate contains phenols, antioxidant chemicals that are also present in red wine, and by now everyone who is interested in living longer knows that antioxidants prevent fat-like substances in the blood from oxidizing and clogging the arteries.

"It's raising a hypothesis that, if true, would bring cheer to those who like chocolate," said Dr. I-Min Lee, an epidemiology professor at Harvard who led the research. I am indeed one of those.

<u>Eating Nuts</u>:

Fortunately I have been in love with all kinds of nuts since I was a young boy in North Carolina. During the great depression, shaking pecan trees and harvesting the nuts was a wonderful, but sometimes risky way to make extra money for things I needed.

I shook the trees for one half of the harvested nuts and sold my shares for ten cents a pound to the local grocery chain. During the fall of the year I easily made eight to ten dollars on a weekend. At that time ten cents would get me into the Saturday movies. The extra money helped pay for my school clothing and supplies.

I started eating pecans then and have never stopped. Recently I also read in Jean Carper's weekly column, "Eat Smart," that nuts may lower blood cholesterol. Her column, which appears in *USA Weekend* and comes in our local Sunday newspaper, reported that Harvard researchers released a study suggesting nuts may also save you from a deadly heart attack. "Among 22,000 physicians tracked for 12 years, those who ate the most nuts had the fewest deaths from heart disease, regardless of all the other factors, such as exercise, high blood pressure and alcohol use." Lead researcher, Christine M. Albert, M.D., speculates that a type of fat in nuts, alpha-linolenic acid, may help prevent "ventricular fibrillation," a heart rhythm disturbance that causes 250,000 sudden deaths each year.

I could be living proof of this study. I have lower than average cholesterol, no heart attacks and no ventricular fibrillation. For my part I'll just keep on cracking nuts and drinking black or green tea with flavonoids, the same stuff that's in red wine, while continuing to take a beta-blocker. To my knowledge, herbal teas don't have the same good stuff.

Vitamins and Food Supplements:

As mentioned in an earlier chapter, I first became aware of vitamins when one of my associates had a heart attack. At the time he was just forty-five. After several weeks of recuperating he returned to work with all kinds of news on health, vitamins and food supplements. It was apparent that while in the hospital he had done a lot of research on how to be free of additional heart problems and to stay on the top side of the grass.

He strongly recommended that I read *Prevention Magazine*, a publication devoted to preventing diseases by eating the right foods. I thought I was very healthy and I ignored his advice except for taking vitamins E and C. I decided my associate was going a little overboard when he started eating sunflower seeds and rose hips.

About that time Dr. Linus Pauling, winner of the Nobel Peace Prize and the Nobel Prize in Chemistry, began to show up in the news touting the benefits of mega doses of Vitamin C. The vitamin, he said in his book, "Vitamin C and The Common Cold", was like a miracle substance that would prevent colds as well as flu and cancer. He suggested a daily dose of 500mg of Vitamin C, though he took 18,000mg a day. The standard recommended daily dose on multivitamin bottles is 60mg though that is currently under review by the National Institutes of Health.

Now everybody is getting on the bandwagon, even the Japanese are beginning to add "C" to cola.

The news media have picked up on the ratings value of writing about health like they descended on OJ and Monica. Apparently they discovered everyone, including me, was striving to live the eternal life.

I also found that many of my business friends, who were heads of research for several major pharmaceutical companies, were taking daily doses of Vitamin E, C and a multivitamin containing all sorts of good stuff from A to Z. They hoped the concoctions would return them to their younger and healthier days. They, like Ponce de Leon, were still searching for the Fountain of Youth.

Over time, I watched my own associate's health improve remarkably. It was then that I confirmed it was time to change my attitude.

I preface my own regimen of vitamins with the caveat that I don't believe this stuff is an instant cure for anything. I firmly believe that, as with pharmaceutical drugs, there's a loading time necessary for the body to make any changes in its metabolism. And even then some of them can be highly questionable.

For example CoQ-10 was highly recommended by a person on the Internet as having helped her lick her atrial fibrillation. She was very convincing, but I later learned she was also an agent for the makers. Regardless of that, I decided to give it a try even though it seemed to be expensive. While it may only be psychological it makes me feel as though I have more stamina than I had prior to its introduction to my regimen. It could be the placebo effect. It also helps to know that CoQ-10 was developed in Japan. After all, to repeat once again, Japan seems to have a world-wide lock on healthy hearts. In any case a recent national study is touting CoQ-10 as an assist in keeping healthy gums.

Presently I'm combining my doctor's regimen of prescribed drugs, 12 and a half mg once a day of Toprol ® (metoprolol, a beta-blocker), 100 mg twice a day of flecainide acetate, (though I've recently learned from talking to Dr. William Miles in May of 2000 that flecainide often converts atrial fibrillation to atrial flutter) and 81mg once a day of aspirin, with my own concoction of the following vitamins: a multivitamin/multimineral A to Z....as well as 400 IU units of E...500 mg C USP...150 mg CoQ-10....150 mg Cellmins Magnesium. This one, like CoQ-10, is touted to strengthen the heart muscle.

For the time being, that's it. If they're indeed the devil's potion, so be it. I'll keep taking them unless my cardiologist finds something that works better. This combination helps me believe I'm doing something good for myself, and apparently I'm suffering no peculiar side effects - as I did in the case of grapefruit.

As I said earlier, an added incentive to my quest for better health is my old vitamin enriched associate who retired in good health at 75 and at the time of his last Christmas card was 86 and still going strong.

<u>Tricks of the Medical Trade</u>:

Presuming the readers remember the very beginning of this one man "clinical trial", they might specifically recall how, on the day and time of discovery, my doctor massaged a nerve that runs vertically down my neck just under the angle of my jaw. He did this in short intervals for about five minutes. The flutter stopped and my heart returned to sinus rhythm (normal).

Later, I decided his maneuver was like a miracle and I needed to research it more. I might add he didn't explain at the time just what he was doing to me and my search didn't prove successful till I purchased a copy of the recently printed *Merck Manual*. This book was written for the general public. Since the beginning of time Merck has published a widely used and very well respected technical manual for physicians. Over the years I've had copies of various editions and on many occasions they helped me in my pharmaceutical consulting practice, though most of the time the information I wanted to research was way over my head.

Fortunately, this home edition is written in simple and easily understood language expressively for the layman and I believe every household should have one, especially those without Internet access. Surprisingly this large reference manual sells for just $29.95. Under atrial fibrillation I found a reference to the vagal maneuver. It described the same technique my doctor used on me. However, the reference clearly pointed out that only a qualified doctor should perform it. Otherwise it could be dangerous. One might confuse the carotid artery with the vagus nerve and pressing that could interrupt the flow of blood to the brain.

I was happy to find under the same subject a couple of other simple procedures I could use that might help eliminate my A-fib or stop it soon after it starts.

The second one seemed a bit funny, but I decided the next time my heart was in A-fib I would try it no matter how ridiculous it made me feel.

It suggested one engage in a straining effort as though one were constipated. That would be easy, I've had lots of experience with this one.

The third sounded just as peculiar, but as I said earlier, who cares if it works.

While in A-fib, the sufferer should douse his face in ice cold water and hold it there for a while. Instead of the cold water routine, I've obtained two pliable ice packs that are commonly used for injured muscles which I keep in the freezer and when an A-fib starts, apply them to my face, forehead and back of the neck until it subsides.

And last, but not least, I cough heavily. I suppose the theory here is that coughing jolts the heart enough for it to reenter sinus rhythm, its normal pace.

Any or all of these done together or separately seemed to work, but mostly I do them all together.

I feel the combination of these tricks of the trade, vitamins, drugs and exercise definitely interrelate and have cut my time in atrial fib from as many as three a week to just two a year and the duration of the episodes has been cut from 7 to 15 hours to 1 to 5 hours.

I calculate this to be about a 90% gain when measuring the time one could be exposed to a stroke. This translates into a major improvement from when I was taking drugs alone.

And above all, according to Philip E. Ross in the August 9, 1999 issue of *Forbes*, "You had better educate yourself about the latest medical breakthroughs, because there is a good chance your internist has neg-

GOD HELPS THOSE WHO HELP THEMSELVES

lected to do so.

"In medicine 85% to 90% of doctors operate alone, or in small groups that at most share calls. How can they keep up with the 1,300 medical articles published every day?

"What's a patient to do? Take charge of your health care, seek second opinions - and make sure someone you trust second-guesses your doctors when you can no longer do so yourself."

Mr. Ross is indeed on the money. Over the last three years I have done research in some 20 medical books, read hundreds of medical journals, an equal number of national and international newspaper health care writers, innumerable Internet health care articles, exchanged e-mails with over 200 A-fib sufferers via the Internet, and consulted with world class cardiologists in the field of arrhythmia health care.

My library on atrial fibrillation/flutter is voluminous. All this, to a very large extent, is what made this published work possible. During this research effort I've often asked myself how can any doctor have time to treat his patients when subjecting himself to this kind of research on a single disease? I personally believe they can't possibly do it and have time for anything else.

My wife jokingly says that with all the above regimen I should live to be as old as Methuselah.

XVIII

RAINBOWS
IN OUR FUTURE

In the 21st Century, I believe the medical and surgical professional researchers are on the threshold of many exciting and newly improved heart-assist devices. The pharmaceutical companies will also make new discoveries in medications that may very well cure the heart of its irregular antics.

I was reassured that this was indeed the case after talking with Dr. Brian McGovern and his colleagues, Dr. Jeremy Ruskin and Dr. David Keane, all of whom hold prominent appointments, dealing exclusively with arrhythmias, at Massachusetts General Hospital/ Harvard Medical School in Boston.

In May 2000, Dr. McGovern chaired a "Clinical Tutorial on New Class III Antiarrhythmic Drugs" at the North American Society of Pacing and Electrophysiology

21st Annual Scientific Sessions in Washington, D.C. Dr. Ruskin was the Presenter of "Implications of Primary and Secondary Prevention Trials for ICD Use in Clinical Practice" at this same Annual Scientific Sessions.

Dr. McGovern told me, "It is great to see the interest that is developing in atrial fibrillation as manifested by the frequency of articles in the press, TV, and on the Web. As you know, atrial fibrillation is very common, often very troublesome for patients, and associated in some individuals with a risk of congestive heart failure or stroke.

"There are new therapies which are certainly much better than what we had in the past but are still limited. It will be interesting to watch over the next number of years with the research effort that is going on now whether the pharmaceutical industry, device industry, catheter manufacturers, and others working in collaboration with investigative physicians can devise more satisfactory therapies than what are currently available.

"There is quite a lot of new work being done now in mapping the initiating events for fibrillation within the pulmonary veins which drain the blood from the lungs to the left atrium. It turns out that in some individuals, particularly younger patients with normal hearts, that extra beats within (atrial tissue extending into) the veins coming from the lungs actually initiate atrial fibrillation. In some individuals, it's now been possible to identify these areas and using radiofrequency techniques to ablate them. This is a much safer approach than linear ablation within the left atrium which, as you know, carries some risk of stroke."

As I said in an earlier chapter, I was not convinced that radiofrequency ablation was the technique of choice, but observing the speed of development and new confirmations as late as May 2000, has convinced me that it is indeed a procedure that merits my strong reconsideration.

For example, Dr. Francis E. Marchlinski, of the Hospital of the University of Pennsylvania, reported in the February 2000 issue of the *Journal of the American College of Cardiology* that his high rate of success with ablation spans all age groups including octogenarians. To me this confirms the rate of speed in which researchers and doctors are moving to use ablation to cure or improve this condition.

Dr. Marchlinski said, "The discovery of the triggers for atrial fibrillation being located in the pulmonary vein will undoubtedly be recognized as one of the principle discoveries that will allow us to cure this disease."

In confirming these latest developments, I once again contacted Dr. William Miles, formerly with the Krannert Institute at the Indiana University Medical Center and now with the SouthwestHeart Group in Fort Myers, Florida, and Dr. Jeremy Ruskin at Massachusetts General Hospital and they assured me that radiofrequency ablation for flutter in many cases can be highly effective.

At Miles's suggestion I contacted Dr. Jeffrey E. Olgin, Assistant Professor of Medicine at the Krannert Institute, who feels that ablation is the first line of treatment for atrial flutter because it is well understood by doctors and it does not respond particularly well to drug therapy. He added that some patients, after being ablated for flutter, need to remain on flecainide or a like drug to control their fibrillation, which in some patients occurs after ablating the flutter.

In the chapter on the Curative Maze Procedure, I mentioned the Cleveland Clinic as a leading cardiac surgery hospital. Just before this book went to press, on NBC's May 18, 2000 edition of Nightly News with Tom Brokaw, the hospital was featured as a nationally pre-eminent heart center in their series of the "Best Hospitals in America" for various medical specialities. During the Brokaw report one of Cleveland Clinic's leading surgeons stressed that their team care and the lack of direct renumeration by the patient played a major role in their success.They are all paid employees of the Cleveland Clinic.

This presentation reminded me that currently Cleveland Clinic is not only rated the best hospital for cardiac care, but has been in this position, according to *U.S. News and World Report* and the National Opinion Research Center, for the last five years. They hold this rank out of 1631 tertiary care centers in the United States.

For information for the readers of this book, the other top ten rated hospitals in this category, which are by no means less than excellent, are: Mayo Clinic, Massachusetts General Hospital, Brigham and Women's Hospital, Duke University Medical Center, Johns Hopkins Hospital, Texas Heart Institute-St. Luke's Episcopal Hospital, Emory University Hospital, Stanford University Hospital, and Barnes-Jewish Hospital.

I predict it will be a scientist in a research group, and most likely a molecular biologist, or an electrophysiologist from one of these hospital who will expand our knowledge of the cell membrane components that participate in the generation and propagation of electrical impulses (the spark that does it all). With this information, biotechnology companies will be able to target specific proteins that are abnormal and create drugs to do their job. Most of this will be a consequence of the June 2000 announcement of the human genome map.

I firmly believe newer development companies such as Thermo Cardiosystems with their HeartMate, Abiomed with AbioCor which are creating heart assist apparatuses (LVAS, left ventricular assist systems), and Cardima, with their mapping process, are on the right track.

Abiomed's AbioCor has taken the final step of

transmitting electricity through the patient's skin, sending the current from an external battery to an internal wire much like that of an automobile coil. In the next decade I believe they will have an apparatus that will totally replace the damaged heart.

Until recently, in my mind, it has seemed as if they are searching for the needle in the haystack, though time seems to be on the side of those who are not currently suffering from very frequent symptomatic bouts of fibrillation or chronic atrial fibrillation.

As recently as mid-1999, the July 12 edition of *U.S. News and World Report,* had a story, "On Improved Diagnoses," by Jennifer Couzin. She described how scientists are developing new techniques in magnetic resonance, or MRI, that will be a vast improvement over the fuzzy imaging of echocardiograms, thereby resulting in better diagnoses.

The pharmaceutical industry will continue to search for a curative drug to replace those that now have only temporary effect.

As late as October of 1999 the FDA sent a letter of approval to Pfizer for Tikosyn® (dofetilide), an antiarrhythmic for conversion of chronic atrial fibrillation to normal sinus rhythm and for maintenance of sinus rhythm in patients who have been converted from AF. This is the first new antiarrhythmic drug in 10 years. It has been released by the FDA with the caveat that doctors must take a training course in the administering of this drug because of its potential lethal side effects. As I said earlier, in the beginning flecainide was responsible for several deaths with patients who had underlying heart disease. Since I am personally on a low dose of flecainide, I am grateful that I have been thoroughly tested for underlying problems and have been found to have none.

Proctor and Gamble was prepared to release a new drug, Stedicor®, for the same treatment, though its release has been delayed by the FDA for the time being.

CV Therapeutics, Inc., of Palo Alto, California, announced on May 16, 2000, that it had successfully completed the first segment of its Phase II clinical program of CVT-510, a potential new drug for the management of atrial arrhythmias. As a result of these data the company is now progressing into Phase III clinical trials.

There is no doubt in my mind that there are several other companies poised to announce new antiarrhythmic drugs in the near future.

While I don't believe they're representing them to be curative drugs, it's an indication of the continuing search for such drugs to replace those that now have only a temporary effect. We patients will more happily continue to play the role of guinea pig, while hoping for the cure.

Fortunately, more serious AF sufferers still have the invasive procedures like radiofrequency ablation or the maze procedure that are here now and the use of medical devices such as the new cardiac rhythm management device developed by Vitatron of Medtronics, Inc. As recently as May 3, 2000, this device is being used outside of the United States and, according to Dr. Jeffrey Olgin, is about to be approved for use in this country. It is a very sophisticated device with ways to prevent atrial fibrillation, ways to terminate atrial fibrillation without a shock and the ability to give a shock initiated by the patient. It is not a cure-all and is not for everybody. More specific information about this device can be obtained from Medtronics' Web Page - www.medtronic.com/news/articles.

For the common run of patients, like myself, it appears that open heart surgery is a bit drastic, although Dr. Cox is currently working on a procedure that would not require opening the chest to get to the heart. To date (mid-2000) he has performed this newer, less invasive maze procedure on 65 patients who have certain physical characteristics which are compatible with this procedure.

At the 1999 American Heart Association Conference in Atlanta he reported on 50 of these 65 patients. He said he's had as high a degree of success with this approach as he has had with the full blown operation. The long-term recurrence of atrial fibrillation was equally low and fewer patients required pacemakers following the minimally invasive procedure.

RAINBOWS IN OUR FUTURE

For the worth of it all, early in the book I presented two letters - one (on page 121) from a patient who has had the more invasive maze operation performed by Dr. Cox and one (on page 62) from a patient who has had the radiofrequency ablation procedure. Both people seem to be very determined to escape the drug regimens that they had been on for many years without success. The letters speak for themselves.

Recently, Dr. Mullane has advised me that clinicians and scientists have presented advances at the November 1999 annual Scientific Sessions of the American Heart Association. Work is in progress evaluating: 1) how atrial fibrillation develops; 2) how established fibrillation impacts the structure and electrophysiology of the heart; 3) how atrial tissue can be mapped in the pulmonary veins and ablative procedures in the veins be improved; 4) how atrial fibrillation can be better prevented and managed with current pharmaceutical, surgical, dietary and device therapies; and 5) how clinicians can focus on improving quality of life for the patient with atrial fibrillation.

In hopeful anticipation of these new scientific developments, I will continue my regimen of less stress, better diet and vitamin supplements, regular daily walks and my current medications, as long as this combination continues to reduce the number of episodes per year (from 3 a week to 2 a year) and the amount of negative time spent in a fib (from 7 to 15 hours to 1 to 5 hours).

I fervently believe that most people who suffer with this elusive and almost ephemeral mystery can do the same if they, with the right doctor (one who will spend as much time with you on the third and fourth visits as on the first), participate in their own health care and follow the disciplines that this malady requires. Why, I ask myself, should anyone totally put a life into the hands of someone you hardly know whether they be doctor, priest or scientist?

Last, but certainly not least, is the Internet and its multiplicity of excellent medical web sites. It clearly opens the world up with medical information the patient needs to help make informed decisions.

As I've said repeatedly throughout this work, if patients help themselves, their doctors can help them better and they will surely see rainbows in the future.

GLOSSARY

This Glossary is intended to make clearer some terms used in this book. For more precise definitions, check with your library's medical dictionary.

ABLATION - A procedure that destroys heart tissue using radiofrequency or DC current, usually performed through a catheter to the heart from the arm or groin. Its purpose is to stop chaotic electrical impulses.

ACCESSORY PATHWAY - A supplementary pathway which allows electrical impulses to go directly from the atria to the ventricles.

ADRENERGIC AF - A type of atrial fibrillation associated with excessive adrenaline that originates with the sympathetic response of the nervous system.

AMIODARONE - A medication which can have substantial toxicity and is used primarily to suppress ventricular arrhythmias, but may also be used to suppress atrial fibrillation.

ANTIARRHYTHMIC - A medication used to control or convert heart rhythm by altering the electrophysiology of cardiac cells.

ANTICOAGULANT - Suppresses, delays or inhibits clotting of blood. Coumadin® and heparin are most commonly prescribed.

ARRHYTHMIA - Heart rhythms which vary from the normal rhythm of the heart beat.

ATRIA - The two upper chambers of the heart which receive blood from the body (right atrium) and lungs (left atrium) and deliver it to the right and left ventricles.

ATRIAL DEFIBRILLATOR - An experimental devise implanted near the heart that delivers minuscule electrical shocks to the heart to terminate atrial arrhythmias.

ATRIAL DILATATION - Enlargement of the atria.

ATRIAL FIBRILLATION (AF) - The normal, regular contractions of the atria are replaced by rapid, irregular twitchings of the muscular wall. The disorganized frequency of fibrillation ranges from 350 to 600 quivers per minute. The ventricles respond irregularly to atrial excitations and a ventricular tachycardia frequently exists in untreated patients. The pulse rate in the wrist can reflect the rate of ventricular contractions, but the patient can not perceive the atrial rate without the aid of an electrocardiogram.

ATRIAL FLUTTER - The atria has rapid, regular contractions usually at rates between 240 and 350 beats per minute. The ventricles do not respond to each atrial excitation. Typically the ventricular rate is one half the atrial rate (2:1 block) but ratios for the block can even be 5 or 6:1. Chronic atrial flutter often converts to atrial fibrillation.

ATRIAL MAPPING - Using electrophysiolocal techniques to trace the movement of electrical impulses in the atria.

ATRIAL PACEMAKER - A low voltage electrical stimuli to the atria.

ATRIAL TACHYCARDIA - A type of atrial arrhythmia from three or more electrical complexes with rates above 100 beats per minute (BPM).

ATRIAL THROMBUS - A clot that forms in the atria.

AV NODAL ABLATION - A specialized catheter delivers electrical energy to interrupt or curtail the flow of electrical impulses that moves from the top to the bottom of the heart. After this procedure, a pacemaker is inserted to maintain regular ventricular beats.

AV NODE - The area between the atria and the ventricles where electrical impulses moving from the top to the bottom of the heart momentarily slow down to allow time for the atria to pump blood into the ventricles.

BETA-BLOCKER - Medications that reduce heart rate and the work load of the heart by blocking the beta adrenergic sympathetic responses. They are used to treat arrhythmias, hypertension, angina pectoris, and tremor and to prevent heart attacks and migraine.

BRADYARRHYTHMIA - When the heart rhythm is slow and irregular.

BRADYCARDIA - When the heart beats 60 per minute or less.

CALCIUM-CHANNEL BLOCKER - Medications that work by inhibiting the movement of ions into vascular and cardiac cells. They dilate peripheral arteries and relieve coronary artery spasm and are used to treat

hypertension and angina pectoris. Some calcium-channel blockers such as diltiazem and verapamil can slow ventricular tachycardia in patients with atrial flutter or fibrillation.

CARDIAC CATHETERIZATION - A specialized technique that uses catheters and dye to observe the coronary arteries that supply the heart with blood.

CARDIOVERSION, ELECTRICAL - A procedure that uses an electrical charge to return the heart to sinus rhythm (normal).

CARDIOVERSION, PHARMACOLOGICAL - A procedure that uses drugs to return the heart to sinus rhythm (normal).

CATHETER ABLATION - A procedure using specialized catheters to direct electrical energy in order to destroy heart tissue which is causing an arrhythmia.

CEREBRAL VASCULAR ACCIDENT (CVA) - Describes a stroke.

CHRONIC ATRIAL FIBRILLATION - This is a persistent form of atrial fibrillation which usually occurs in patients with cardiovascular disease. Patient symptoms and complaints are related to ventricular tachycardia, embolization, decreased cardiac output and anxiety.

COUMADIN® - See Warfarin and INR (International Normalized Ratio)

DIGITALIS - A medication that increases the force of the heart and slows the rate.

DILTIAZEM® - A calcium channel blocker

ECHOCARDIOGRAM - The ultrasound pictures of the heart.

ELECTROPHYSIOLOGIST (EP) - A cardiologist with expertise in the electrical phenomena associated with cardiac arrhythmias and in the means to treat these disorders.

EMBOLISM - A dislodged blood clot, cancer cell, fat or air bubble which obstructs the flow of blood.

FAMILIAL AF - A rare type of atrial fibrillation linked to genetic defects.

FLAVONOID - Chemicals of plant origin which may have beneficial effects on cancer, cardiovascular disease, and immune system function. The antioxidants found in black and green tea are examples.

FLECAINIDE - An antiarrhythmic drug used to treat both ventricular and atrial arrhythmias. Also know as Tambocor®

HEPARIN - An anticoagulant.

HOLTER MONITOR - A portable EKG system that the patient can wear at home while recording heart rhythms during normal activities.

HYPOTENSION - Low blood pressure.

HYPERTHYROIDISM - A hypermetabolic state that occurs from an overactive thyroid gland. Atrial fibrillation can be a manifestation of the disease.

INTERNATIONAL NORMALIZED RATIO (INR) - To standardize monitoring of warfarin (Coumadin®) dosing, prothrombin time results are reported as a ratio (INR). The system is based on the use of test reagents that are standardized for activity against an international reference prepared by the World Health Organization. A normal INR is 1.0. The recommended INR for patients receiving warfarin for non-valvular atrial fibrillation is 2.0 - 3.0. An INR of greater than 4.0 is associated with a higher risk of bleeding.

LONE ATRIAL FIBRILLATION - Atrial fibrillation with no identifiable cause or underlying heart disease.

MAZE PROCEDURE - A surgical procedure that cures atrial fibrillation by interrupting the circular wavelets of electrical energy that are typical of this arrhythmia. Strategic placement of multiple incisions in both atria stops the formation of errant electrical impulses and channels the normal electrical impulses in one direction from the top of the heart to the bottom.

NORMAL SINUS RHYTHM (NSR) - The rhythm for heart beats is established by normal electrical pathways.

PACEMAKER - A low voltage electrical device implanted in the patient to cause the heart muscle to contract.

PAROXYSMAL ATRIAL FIBRILLATION - A intermittent type of atrial fibrillation.

PROARRHYTHMIC - Drugs used to control arrhythmias can in a low percentage of patients induce arrhythmias.

GLOSSARY

PROPRANOLOL - A beta-blocker.

PACs - Premature atrial contractions.

PVCs - Premature ventricular contractions.

RHEUMATIC HEART DISEASE - Heart damage can
be a result of rheumatic fever. The heart valves and
myocardium can be affected.

SA NODE - Considered to be the primary pacemaker of
the heart

SOTOLOL - A beta-blocker.

SUPRAVENTRICULAR TACHYCARDIA (SVT) - A
fast and regular rhythm greater than 100 beats per
minute that starts above the ventricles.

TACHYCARDIA - A heart beat greater than 100 beats
per minute.

TRANSIENT ATRIAL FIBRILLATION - Same as
paroxysmal AF.

TRANSIENT ISCHEMIC ATTACKS (TIAs) - Brief
cerebrovascular incidents which can result in temporary

speech or visual disturbances, numbness, weakness or unconsciousness that occurs as a result of blockage of small arteries. Repeated TIAs can lead to dementia.

VAGAL AF - A type of atrial fibrillation believed to be triggered indirectly by an abnormal increase of the activity of the vagus nerve.

VAGUS NERVE - Comprises part of the body's longest pair of cranial nerves and is responsible for many critical functions, among them digestion, speech and swallowing.

VERAPAMIL - A calcium-channel-blocker.

WARFARIN - A drug used as an anticoagulant. Coumadin® is DUPONT'S trademark name.

WOLFF-PARKINSON-WHITE (WPW) SYNDROME
An atrioventricular conduction disorder associated with tachycardia. Usually there are two separate AV conduction pathways. Atrial flutter and fibrillation are common in patients with WPW.

BIBLIOGRAPHY

Altman, Lawrence K., M.D., After 40 Years,
Pacemakers Are Smarter and Safer
New York Times, October 27, 1998

Altman, Lawrence K., M.D., Boy's Death in Surgery is
Lesson on Nonprescription Drug
New York Times, March 17, 1998

Associated Press, Washington dateline, AMA Says
Some Chinese Herbal Remedies Are OK
Glens Falls Post Star, November 11, 1998

Associated Press, Washington, D.C. dateline,
Confusing Drug Names Can Lead to Mistakes
Glens Falls Post Star, November 27, 1998

185

Beware the Hostile Heart
From the *Fort Worth Star-Telegram*
Reprinted in the *Glens Falls Post Star*
September 8, 1998

Brink, Susan, The Drugs of Choice
U.S. News & World Report
November 16, 1998

Brody, Jane, Pass the Wine and Olive Oil, and Other
Lessons From Crete
New York Times, February 10, 1998

Brody, Jane, Dietary Supplements May Test
Consumers' Health
New York Times, September 22, 1998

Brody, Jane, Alternative Medicine Makes Inroads, But
Watch Out for Curves
New York Times, April 28, 1998

Burton, Thomas M., An HMO Checks Up On Its
Doctors' Care and Is Disturbed Itself
Wall Street Journal, July 8, 1998

Cohen, Jay S., MD,The One Size Dose
Does Not Fit All
Newsweek, December 6, 1999

Couzin, Jennifer, Improved Diagnoses, Focusing on
the Heart as a Moving Target
U.S. News & World Report, July 12, 1999

Cox, James, L. MD, et al Current Status of the Maze
Procedure for the Treatment of Atrial Fibrillation
Seminars in Thoracic and Cardiovascular Surgery
January, 2000

Editorial: Removal of Posicor an
Alarming Sign for FDA
Glens Falls Post Star, June 12, 1998

Educated Seek Alternate Cures,
From the *Washington Post*
Reprinted in the *Glens Falls Post Star,* June 2, 1998

Fried, Stephen, Bad Medicine on Prescription Drugs
Washington Post National, Weekly Edition,
June 8, 1998

Goldstein, Amy, A Lesson in Bedside Manners
Washington Post National, Weekly Edition
October 12, 1998

Goodman, Ellen, Ads Turn Patients into Consumers
Glens Falls Post Star, July 2, 1999

Grady, Denise, As Silent Killer Returns, Doctors
Rethink Tactics to Lower Blood Pressure
New York Times, July 14, 1998

Gugliotta, Guy, A Heart-Stopping Solution
Washington Post National Weekly Edition,
July 12, 1999

Harriman, Jane, A Heart Out of Control
Des Moines Register, Family Home Health Journal

BIBLIOGRAPHY

Hope for Heart Attack Victims
U.S. News & World Report,
July 20, 1998

Jackson, Nancy Beth, Doctors' Warning: Beware of
Herbs' Side Effects
New York Times,
November 17, 1998

Kolata, Gina, Where Marketing and Medicine Meet
New York Times,
February 10, 1998

Lipsyte, Robert, It's Enough to Make You Sick, The
Way Patients Get Treated
New York Times,
Sunday, June 21, 1998

Marchlinski, Francis E., MD,Catheter Ablation
Recommended for Octogenarians with Arrhythmias
Journal of the American College of Cardiology
February, 2000

McCarthy, Patrick M., MD, et al The Cox-Maze
Procedure:The Cleveland Clinic Experience
Seminars in Thoracic and Cardiovascular Surgery,
January, 2000

Neenan, Julia McNamee, Good News for Chocaholics
HealthSCOUT @ Earthlink, August 7, 1999

Neergaard, Lauren, Slicing a Heart to Make It Beat
Glens Falls Post Star, March 29, 1998
(Associated Press)

Novotny, Pamela Patrick, When the Heart Misfires
Reader's Digest, September, 1994

Porter, Roy, The Greatest Benefit to Mankind
Book Review by David Hollinger,
New York Times Book Review, May 13, 1998

Rogers, Adam, Good Medicine on the Web
Newsweek, August 23, 1998

BIBLIOGRAPHY

Ross, Philip E, Help Me, Doctor
Forbes, August 9, 1999

Roth, Katherine, Tea Touted For Heart-Healthy Diet
(Associated Press)
Glens Falls Post Star, July 12, 1999

Sternberg, Steve, Michael DeBakey's Living Legacy
USA Today - Life Section, November 2, 1998

Stolberg, Sheryl, Heart Drug Withdrawn as Evidence
Shows It Could be Lethal
New York Times, June 8, 1998

Stroh, Michael, Unhappy Patients Turn to Online
Doctors
From the *Baltimore Sun*
Reprinted in the *Glens Falls Post Star,* June 2, 1998

Wells, Susan J., Heart Risk Tied to Job Situations
New York Times, April 12, 1998

191

MY HEART, THE DOCTORS and me

Winslow, Ron, Heart Researchers Find Beta-Blockers
of Little Benefit in Improving Survival
Wall Street Journal

Zuger, Abigail, How Grapefruit Juice Makes Some
Pills More Powerful
New York Times, October 7, 1998

Zuger, Abigail, When the Doctor and Patient Need
Couple's Therapy
New York Times, March 31, 1998

WEB PAGES

Note: The relative newness of some Web pages causes constant updating and some of the following Internet addresses may have changed since the printing of this book. If a problem occurs, phone the 800 number of the organization or check your search engine.

American Heart Association
www.americanheart.org

Cardiac Pathways
www.cardiac.com

Cardima - Microcatheter solutions for EP
www.cardima.com/

Case Western Reserve University
www.cwru.edu

Clinical Results - Cardiac Arrhythmias
www.cardiac.com/Pages/inside/clinic/index.html

e medicine
www.emedicine.com

Guidant - Cardiac Rhythm management
www.guidant.com

Harvard Heart Letter
www.harvardhealthpubs.org

Heart Disease News
www..mediconsult.com/

Internet FDA
www..fda.gov/

WEB PAGES

Internet Medical Advise
www.americasdoctor.com
www.cyberdocs.com
www.webmd.com

Johns Hopkins Health Information
www.intelihealth.com

Massachusetts General Hospital
www.mgh.harvard.edu

Mayo Clinic
www.mayohealth.org/

Maze Information -
Terry Palazzo's site and bulletin board
http://members.aol.com/mazern/index.htm
http://members.aol.com/mazern/post.htm

Medscape
www.medscape.com/

Medtronics, Inc.
www.medtronic.com/

Thrive on - Health Letter
www.thriveonline.com

Nature - International Weekly Journal of Science
www.nature.com

Science News Online
www.sciencenews.org

The New England Journal of Medicine
www.nejm.org/

The New York Times - Science Page
www.nytimes.com

The Medical Web Destination Patients Use Most
www.mediconsult.com

WEB PAGES

The Cleveland Clinic foundation
www.ccf.org

Tufts University Diet & Nutrition Letter, 1990
www.thriveonline.com/

UCSF Stanford Health Care
www.med.stanford.edu/shc

University of Kentucky - Chandler Medical Center
www.mc.uky.edu

Virginia Commonwealth University
www.vcu.edu

Washington University in St. Louis
www.wust.edu

U.S. News and World Report
www.usnews.com

MY HEART, THE DOCTORS and me

United States National Library of Medicine
www.ncbi.nlm.nih.gov/

National Institutes of Health
www.nih.gov

Department of Health and Human Services
www.dhhs.gov

BOOKS OF INTEREST

Bitter Pills: Inside the Hazardous World of Drugs
by Stephen Fried
Bantam, New York, New York

Catheter Ablation for Arrhythmias - A Patient's Guide
Health Trend Publishing, P.O. Box 7390
Menlo Park, CA 94026
1-415-462-1881
(Distributed by the Krannert Institute of Cardiology -
Indianapolis, Indiana)

Demanding Medical Excellence
by Michael L. Millenson
The University of Chicago Press

MY HEART, THE DOCTORS and me

The Merck Manual of Medical Information
Home Edition
The Merck Publishing Group, Rahway, New Jersey

University Medical Center
Indianapolis, Indiana
1-800-843-2786

Make Your Medicine Safe
by Dr. Jay S. Cohen
Avon Books

Modern Management of Acute Myocardial Infarction
In The Community Hospital
Edited by
Dr. Jeffrey A. Anderson

RECORDS OF YOUR PERSONAL HISTORY

One of the best ways to help your doctor help you is to maintain an accurate accounting of all incidents of any arrhythmias, <u>when they start,</u> <u>when they stop</u>, and all the drugs you are taking. It's important to list the milligrams (mg), the intervals and daily amounts. The pages following the list of drug names can be used for this purpose.

*****

To help you with the names of drugs, I have listed the drugs I have been taking or have mentioned in this book. The registered trademark of the drug's original manufacturer is given first, the generic (World Health Organization's) name is second, and the manufacturer's name is last.

Cordarone® - amiodarone - Wyeth Ayerst Pharmaceuticals

Betapace® - sotalol - Berlex Laboratories

Cardizem® - diltiazem - Hoechst Marion Roussel

Coumadin® - warfarin sodium - DuPont Pharmaceutical Company

Cozaar® - losartan - E.I. DuPont deNemours & Company

Ethmozine® - moricizine - Roberts Pharmaceutical Corporation

Inderal® - propranolol - Wyeth Ayerst Pharmaceuticals

Isoptin® - verapamil - Knoll Laboratories

Lanoxin® - digoxin - Glaxo Wellcome, Inc.

Norpace® - disopyramide phosphate - G. D. Searle & Company

Neo-Synephrine® - phenylephrine hydrochloride - Sanofi Pharmaceuticals, Inc.

Pepcid® - famotidine - Merck & Company, Inc.

Premarin® - conjugated estrogens - Wyeth Ayerst Pharmaceuticals

Propulsid® - cisapride - Janssen Pharmaceuticals

Robitussin® - guaifenesin - A. H. Robins Company

Rythmol® - propafenone - Knoll Laboratories

Sectral® - acebutolol - Wyeth Ayerst Pharmaceuticals

Stedicor® - azimilide - Proctor & Gamble Pharmaceuticals

Tagamet® - cimetidine - SmithKline Beecham Pharmaceuticals

RECORDS OF YOUR PERSONAL HISTORY

Tambocor® - flecainide - 3 M Pharmaceuticals

Tenormin - atenolol - AstraZeneca LP

Tikosyn® - dofetilide - Pfizer

Toprol® - metoprolol - AstraZeneca LP

Zantac® - ranitidine - Glaxo Wellcome, Inc.

RECORDS OF PERSONAL HISTORY

RECORDS OF PERSONAL HISTORY

RECORDS OF PERSONAL HISTORY

RECORDS OF PERSONAL HISTORY

RECORDS OF PERSONAL HISTORY